Acupuncture for Stroke Rehabilitation

Three Decades of Information from China

Dear Patty Doyle

Hoy Ping Yee Chan,
L.Ac., O.M.D.
et al.

Published by:
BLUE POPPY PRESS
A Division of Blue Poppy Enterprises, Inc.
5441 Western Ave., Suite 2
Boulder, CO 80301
www.bluepoppy.com

First Edition, June 2006

ISBN 1-891845-35-7
LCCN #2006925991

Cover & Page design: Eric J. Brearton

COMP Designation: Original work

10 9 8 7 6 5 4 3 2 1

Printed at National Hirschfeld, Denver, CO on Acid-free paper and Soy Inks

Dedication

This book is dedicated to the publishers of and contributors to those Chinese medical journals covering the application of acupuncture to stroke rehabilitation over the past 30 years. Additionally, it was written in honor of all the dedicated health care practitioners serving his or her patients recovering from stroke, a leading cause of neurological disability worldwide.

There is a well-known Chinese saying:

"The healer has the heart of a parent."

The caring heart of a health care practitioner is no less crucial than know-how and skills

Foreword

I have known Hoy Ping Yee Chan for nearly 25 years. I was one of her fledgling students. Later, I became a colleague and friend, and, nearly a decade ago, I worked with her on her first publication, *Window of Health: Ocular Diagnosis and Periocular Acupuncture*. Through the years, Dr. Chan has remained an exceptional role model for many of us as we have grown in our professional capacity. For a select few, she represents what we have wanted to become as professionals. Dr. Chan has influenced thousands of people with her gentle spirit, bright laugh, and genuine excitement regarding Chinese medicine. She is a dedicated clinician, teacher, and healer as well as an excellent ambassador for our medicine.

I was very much encouraged when Dr. Chan first spoke with me about writing a book on the traditional Chinese medicine (TCM) approach to treating stroke. As her former student, I knew she was meticulous and would enthusiastically dedicate herself to such an undertaking. Consequently, the degree of research and inquiry that has gone into this edition has taken years to compile and organize. The text has gone through several drafts, each successively expanding and refining the presentation from the previous one. It has been a labor of love for Dr. Chan and will prove to be a blessing for practitioners of TCM as well as for those who will benefit therapeutically from her work.

I am honored that Dr. Chan has asked me to write the Foreword for her second book. I am a strong believer in the use of acupuncture for stroke rehabilitation. I have seen its effectiveness in a variety of settings. My first experience was in Chongqing, China, in 1985. At that time, the talk around the hospital was regarding an elderly man whose two sons had carried him on a stretcher for two days from a remote village to the TCM hospital where I was working. He had had a stroke and, although relatively stable, was suffering from hemiplegia. Once admitted, he underwent stroke rehabilitation at the hospital using primarily acupuncture therapy. In little more than a month, this elderly man walked out of the hospital and, with the aid of his sons, walked back to his village. To my eyes, this was a remarkable recovery but not to those in China to whom it was an everyday occurrence. In my mind, this one instance stands out above all others as revealing the efficacy of the use of acupuncture for stroke rehabilitation.

I have known of acupuncture for stroke victims being used in nursing homes, hospices, in acupuncture school teaching clinics, and in private homes. It is currently not available in most hospitals, mostly I believe, because of insurance and liability issues. This obstacle has effectively denied care to tens of thousands who might otherwise have significantly benefitted from this therapy. It is imperative that acupuncture becomes more widely employed for the rehabilitation of stroke victims, and I believe that this book has the potential to greatly influence our current thoughts and protocols regarding treatment of stroke. It is for this reason that I am honored to be part of a growing body of awareness in complementary therapies that is strongly influencing our current Western health care system.

Alex Holland, M.Ac., L.Ac.
President of the Asian Institute of Medical Studies in Tucson, AZ
Faculty member of the Program in Integrative Medicine at the University of Arizona Medical School
Author of *Voices of Qi:An Introductory Guide to Traditional Chinese Medicine*
August 20, 2005

Editor's Preface

This book is primarily a collection of research abstracts on the acupuncture treatment of stroke in the People's Republic of China during the last 30 years. This research has been compiled, abstracted, and translated by a team of individuals gathered together and coordinated by Dr. Hoy Ping Yee Chan of Seattle, WA. This material has then been supplemented by Dr. Chan's own studies and many years experience in the treatment of stroke by acupuncture and its related modalities. The treatments contained in this book address both the acute, emergency treatment of stroke and the treatment of its many sequelae during the recuperative and rehabilitative stages. As for the purpose for the compilation of this book, I will let Dr. Chan explain that in her preface which follows. However, this book is meant for students and practitioners of acupuncture and Chinese medicine as well as Western MDs and researchers interested in the acupuncture treatment of this all too common condition.

This book uses the standard Chinese medical translational terminology developed by Nigel Wiseman *et al.,*. as found in his and Feng Ye's *A Practical Dictionary of Chinese Medicine* (Paradigm Publications, Brookline, MA, 1998). In those few instances where we have deviated from that standard, we have noted those deviations in the endnotes of the first chapter in which they appear. All channel acupoints are identified by the World Health Organization (WHO) standard acupoint alpha-numeric nomenclature, however, with the following differences: Lu for LU, St for ST, Sp for SP, Ht for HT, Bl for UB, Ki for KI, Per for HE, TB for TE, and Liv for LV. Points on the conception vessel are prefaced by CV, and points on the governing vessel are prefaced by GV. For extra-channel acupoints, we have used the identification system found in *Acupuncture: A Comprehensive Text* compiled by the Shanghai College of Traditional Chinese Medicine and translated and edited by John O'Connor and Dan Bensky (Eastland Press, Seattle, 1995). All Chinese medicinal identifications are based on Bensky *et al.*'s, *Chinese Herbal Medicine: Materia Medica*, 3rd edition (Eastland Press, Seattle, 2004). Chinese medicinals first appear in Pinyin in italic followed by their Latin pharmacological nomenclature in parentheses.

This book is the most comprehensive account of the acupuncture treatment of stroke available in English, and Blue Poppy Press is honored to be able to present this material to

English language readers and researchers. We are also honored to be able to introduce my long-time friend Dr. Chan to a larger reading audience. We hope and trust that this book helps alleviate the suffering and disability of many of those struck down by this illness since I know of no better person to spearhead this project than Dr. Chan.

Bob Flaws, Managing Editor
Blue Poppy Press
February 1, 2006

Chief Compiler's Preface

Cerebral vascular accident (CVA) or stroke is the most common cause of neurological damage affecting the elderly. It results from oxygen depravation to nerve tissues because of arterial occlusion or brain hemorrhage. The location and severity of the stroke determines the degree of loss of function, and stroke can also lead to death. The usual Western medical approach to stroke rehabilitation is to prescribe approximately eight weeks of physical therapy to aid in recovery. After that, patients are usually left on their own to do the best they can. This not only results in a much longer recovery time but may even impede recovery because, without help, muscles become increasingly weak and atrophied. Patients' quick loss of cardiovascular and muscular fitness and problems with balance all contribute to a pattern of decreased activity which impacts function, independence, and quality of life. This is not only a tragedy for the patients but also for their families and society at large. Hence stroke rehabilitation is not just a medical problem but also a social and economic problem. It is this situation that has led me to the creation of this book.

The condition of stroke has been addressed by Chinese medicine for at least 2,000 years. Symptoms of stroke are recorded in the oldest and most famous Chinese medical text, the *Nei Jing (Inner Classic)*. Many clinical studies in China and other countries have demonstrated that acupuncture can help stroke survivors recover quicker and more completely. Unfortunately, this effective treatment method is still not widely accepted in the developed world. In my experience, very few Western physicians refer stroke patients to acupuncturists. Additionally, many medical insurance providers do not pay for the acupuncture treatment of stroke. Such barriers prevent stroke patients from receiving the help that acupuncture can offer. In more than 20 years of practice in the U.S., the majority of my stroke patients have come for acupuncture rehabilitation many years after the onset of their stroke, long after their condition has become chronic. I find it very sad to see them having gone without effective acupuncture treatment early in their stroke recovery, since this is the most important time for effective treatment. As a consequence, their condition is markedly deteriorated, and they have lost the best window of opportunity for receiving improvement from acupuncture.

There are many different acupuncture techniques for treating stroke, and the choice of the most effective of these to use needs to be determined on an individual basis. Actually, the most important factor is the time at which the patient begins to receive acupuncture treatments. The rule is the sooner treatments start, the better. As soon as the patient's acute condition is stable, it is time to start acupuncture. Such an early start increases acupuncture's effectiveness and long-lasting clinical results. The promotion of such early adoption of acupuncture post-stroke is the main purpose of this book. I hope that sharing the results of the many Chinese clinical trials contained herein will prompt more Western practitioners and their patients to add acupuncture to their program of post-stroke rehabilitation. This review of three decades of use of acupuncture in the People's Republic of China will not only teach the reader specific acupuncture techniques but also places these methods in a Western research-based framework. I encourage stroke survivors themselves, their families, and all health care practitioners to be open-minded and add the use of acupuncture to their armament for treating stroke patients.

Hoy Ping Yee Chan, L.Ac., O.M.D.
National Board Certified in Acupuncture & Chinese Herbology (NCCAOM)
Chinese Acupuncture Center of North Seattle
Mill Creek, Washington, U.S.A.
August 25, 2005

Acknowledgments

This book owes its fruition to an informal group of concerned health care professionals who volunteered their strong support.

Craig Brewer, M.D., recognized the value of acupuncture in stroke rehabilitation, initiated the idea, and gave critical input to the compilation of this book. He wrote Appendix 3: My Experiences with Acupuncture Treating Neurological Conditions.

Alex Holland, M.Ac., L.Ac., offered enthusiastic encouragement which further helped the project gain significant momentum. He also wrote the Foreword.

Peter Lau, M.D., combined his language and medical expertise to present Chinese scientific papers in excerpt form in English in Chapter 7 and compiled some articles in Chapter 6.

Kathleen Michael, Ph.D., RN, CRRN, provided updated information about stroke in America and wrote Appendix 2: Acupuncture in Post-stroke Rehabilitation.

Carole Conlon, L.Ac., compiled some articles in Chapter 5 and Chapter 6. Ms. Conlon also did the final language review on Chapter 1 and 7. She drew all the illustrations for this book.

Stanley Sik Chi Chan, M.S., L.Ac., compiled most of the articles in Chapter 5 and some articles in Chapters 6, and the last article of Chapter 7.

J. Miranda Taylor, L.Ac., M.TCM, did the first language review of Chapters 1-4. Ms. Taylor fine-tuned the presentation style and polished the writing in those chapters. She also compiled Chapter 8.

Vincent Wong, M.S.B.E., M.S.E.E., PE, did editorial revisions and English polishing in Chapters 1-5. He also compiled some articles in Chapter 6.

Yuan-ming Lu, L.Ac., did the first translation of Appendix 1. The Chinese National Standard for Diagnosis of Stroke & Outcomes of Its Treatment

Timberly Link, C.P.A., shared his important thoughts as a caregiver for stroke patients. He wrote Appendix 4.

Many thanks to the above individuals whose generous help was crucial to the successful completion of this book.

Also, special thanks goes to Bob Flaws, L.Ac., who was our editor at Blue Poppy Press.

Above all, I must give thanks and praises to almighty God. It is evident to me that the proactive contribution of the above individuals, each bringing unique expertise and all complementing each other, was not a coincidence but was the result of His divine arrangement. Ultimately, it was by His wisdom, His grace, and His blessing that this work of love was accomplished.

Table of Contents

ONE
Understanding Stroke

Western Medicine & Stroke

Stroke is a rapid onset neurological dysfunction of vascular origin causing focal or
global signs of disturbed cerebral function
lasting more than 24 hours. The aftermath
of stroke in many cases means long periods
of rehabilitation.

Epidemiology

According to the WHO, the annual incidence of stroke is 200 cases per 100,000
persons per year.[1] Stroke is the leading
cause of adult disability in the United
States.[2] Every year, about 750,000
Americans sustain initial cerebrovascular
events, and three-fourths of them are left
with persistent neurological deficits that
impair function.[3] Currently, four million

Americans face the aftermath of stroke.
About one-third of stroke victims have mild
impairments, another third is moderately
impaired, and the reminder is severely
impaired. It is estimated that 16% of
Americans over 65 live with the effects of
stroke.[4] Among the physical impairments
following stroke are gait and balance
deficits[5,6], problems with central neural pat-
terning of movements[7], higher energy
expenditure for ambulation, and increased
risk of falls. These impairments predispose
the chronic stroke patient to an increasingly
sedentary lifestyle, compounding physical
and cardiovascular de-conditioning. The
presence of severe hemiplegia and/or aphasia may prevent the stroke patient from
returning to work. Also, the extreme limita-
tions of movement, particularly in the arm
and hand, force the patient to rely on others

RANKING OF FATALITY RATE OF THE MOST COMMON DISEASES

Rank	U.S.A.	China
First	Heart	Stroke
Second	Cancer	Heart
Third	Stroke	Cancer

for their most basic needs. Therefore, the financial and emotional impact on family members of stroke survivors can be extremely difficult. Thus, any improvements in the functional ability of hemiplegic patients would greatly decrease the time, energy, and cost of caring for them.

Although there has been a decline in stroke mortality in the 20th century, stroke is still the third most common cause of death behind heart disease and cancer.[8] A 1979 survey of fatalities covering 40 Chinese cities showed that the fatality rate of stroke was 24.15%. It was rated as the most common cause of death in China due to disease above heart disease (21.5%) and cancer (20.6%).[9]

Although Dr. Foder mentions some of the current reports which point to the rise of cancer as the leading cause of fatality over heart disease, the reason for the decrease in heart disease mortality is due to the vast improvement in emergency cardiac treatment. In stroke, the range of ages at onset is wide, with most strokes occurring in the seventh decade of life in the U.S. Men tend to have strokes earlier than women, although, overall, there is no significant difference between the sexes. The incidence of stroke of all types is greater the higher the relative weight in both men and women. Serum lipids seem to be related only in the youngest age group studied (50-59 years old). Otherwise, no significant relationship has been observed between serum lipids and the incidence of stroke.[10] According to the latest news from the American Heart Association, cigarette smoking also increases the risk of stroke. Women who smoke half a pack of cigarettes a day have twice the risk of stroke than non-smokers, while women who smoke two packs a day have six times more risk of stroke than nonsmokers.[11] Other risk factors of stroke include a sedentary lifestyle, alco-

hol abuse, cocaine use, hypertension, diabetes, heart disease, carotid artery stenosis, and family history.

Etiology

According to Dr. Robert C. Goiney, the etiology of stroke can be summarized as either due to ischemic infarction or hemorrhagic infarction. Each of these may, in turn, be due to specific causes. For instance, ischemic infarction may be due to arterial thrombosis, arterial emboli, sinovenous thrombosis, or vasculitis, while hemorrhagic infaction may be due to hypertension, traumatic injury, tumor, arterial venous malformation (AVM), aneurysm, and amyloid angiopathy.[12]

Differential diagnosis

Stroke must be differentiated in clinical practice from:

> Primary neoplasm
> Secondary neoplasm
> Infection
> Subdural/epidural hematoma

Nosology

In modern Western medicine, the manifestations of stroke are classified as any of the following five nosologies:

> **1.** Atherothrombosis with brain infarction
> **2.** Cerebral embolus
> **3.** Intracranial hemorrhage. Including subarachnoid hemorrhage (SAH)
> **4.** Others: cerebral arteritis, intracerebral hematoma, malformation, etc.
> **5.** Warning sign: transient ischemic attack (TIA)[13]

However, all true strokes can simply be categorized under two major types: hemorrhagic and ischemic. Approximately 75-80% of all strokes are ischemic.[14] Ischemic strokes are characterized by insufficient blood flow to a portion of the brain, usually the result of occlusion of cerebral arteries (*i.e.*, atherothrombolic stroke, cerebral embolism, etc.). Ischemic stroke can completely cut off blood flow to the region of the brain supplied by the blocked artery. Vascular occlusion can also occur as a result of inflammation of blood vessels (intracranial vasculitis) and high blood viscosity due to excessive numbers of circulating red blood cells (polycythemia), white blood cells (leukemia), platelets, etc.

Hemorrhagic strokes occur when an artery in the brain ruptures or leaks, causing blood to escape into the brain or into the space between the brain and skull. Hypertension and atherosclerosis are leading causes of intracerebral hemorrhagic stroke. Although aneurysms may be congenital, they may be exacerbated or even caused by hypertension. Arterio-venous malformation (AVM) is another congenital blood vessel defect which may cause brain hemorrhage. Subarachnoid hemorrhage (SAH) results from bleeding into the space between the brain and the protective arachnoid membranes. In hemorrhagic stroke, damage occurs in two ways. First, the blood supply is cut off to the parts of the brain beyond the site of the artery rupture. Secondly, the escaped blood forms a mass within the rigid skull, causing increased intracranial pressure, which exerts excessive pressure on the brain. Therefore, massive hemorrhages are devastating, usually fatal. Only about 25% of patients survive from a hemorrhagic stroke accounting for approximately 20% of all strokes.[15]

Diagnosis

The Western medical diagnosis of stroke is based on observation of clinical symptoms, a history of risk factors and the results of diagnostic tests. The diagnosis of stroke is evident when:

1. There is a clear history of loss of specific brain function or functions, *i.e.* a focal neurologic deficit, combined with the exclusion of other diseases, such as tumor.

2. Symptoms come on suddenly or first become apparent upon awakening, especially in a person over 50 years of age with vascular disease or other risk factors for stroke.

Clinical feature of strokes

In **intracranial hemorrhage**, there is abrupt onset of a focal neurological deficit; loss of consciousness or coma, hemiplegia or complete paralysis, signs of a sudden increase in intracranial pressure, including alteration in mental status; headache and vomiting.

Ischemic strokes are characterized by acute or insidious onset of a focal deficit and a history indicative of systemic causes of stroke such as recent myocardial infarction, congestive heart failure, diabetic, polycythemia or atherosclerosis.

Thrombosis, which is most common in the middle-aged and elderly with atherosclerosis, diabetes and hypertension, may develop while the patient is asleep or shortly after awakening or may occur during surgery or after a myocardial infarction (MI).

Embolism occurs at any age, especially among patients with a history of rheumatic heart diseases, endocarditis, post-traumatic valvular disease, myocardial fibrillation and other cardiac dysrythmia. It usually develops rapidly in ten to twenty seconds and without warning.

Transient ischemic attacks (TIAs) are characterized by abrupt onset. Their symptoms are transient, lasting minutes or a few hours at most, and eventually resolve.

Clinical features of Cerebral Vascular Accident (CVA) vary with the artery affected and consequently the portion of the brain it supplies. The severity of damage and the extent of collateral circulation that develops to help the brain compensate for the decreased blood supply affect the symptom picture as well. If the CVA occurs in the left hemisphere, it produces symptoms on the right side of the body. If it occurs in the right hemisphcre, symptoms are on the left side of the body. A CVA that causes cranial nerve damage producing signs of cranial nerve dysfunction on the same side as the hemorrhagic symptoms is usually classified according to the artery affected. For instance:

Middle cerebral artery: aphasia, dysphagia, visual field cuts and hemiparesis on affected side, more severe in the face and arms than in the legs

Carotid artery: weakness, paralysis, numbness, sensory changes and visual disturbances on affected side, altered level of consciousness, bruits, headaches, aphasia and ptosis

Cerebrobasilar artery: weakness on affected side, numbness around lips and mouth, visual field cut, diplopia, poor coordination, dysphagia, slurred speech, dizziness, amnesia and ataxia

Anterior cerebral artery: confusion, weakness and numbness, especially in the leg on affected side, incontinence, loss of coordination, impaired motor and sensory functions and personality changes

Posterior cerebral artery: visual field cuts, sensory impairment, dyslexia, coma, cortical blindness. Usually paralysis is absent.

Laboratory tests[16]

Computed tomography (CT) scan shows evidence of hemorrhagic stroke as well as confirming the presence of aneurysms or arteriovenous malformations immediately, but may not show evidence of thrombotic infarction until 48-72 hours have passed. Transient ischemic attacks may not be visible at all.

Magnetic resonance imaging (MRI) scans provide a clearer three-dimensional picture and can detect smaller injuries in all parts of the brain. They may help identify ischemic or infarcted areas and cerebral swelling. Magnetic resonance imaging is better than CT scan to visualize pathology in the brain stem.

Ultrasonography is especially useful for diagnosing ischemic strokes. It allows the physician to visualize blockages and monitor the blood flow through specific arteries. Of the several types of ultrasound techniques, the most common one is Doppler ultrasound. It is generally used to measure how fast blood moves through the aortic arteries. A higher velocity of blood flow indicates sites where atherosclerotic plaque has narrowed the blood vessels.

Cerebral angiography is an invasive procedure that involves the injection of an opaque contrast solution into the blood stream to produce x-ray image of the blood vessels within the brain. The image shows outlines of blood vessels and pinpoints any occlusion or rupture site. It is especially useful if surgical intervention is indicated.

Lumbar puncture refers to a spinal tap which may be used to identify if there is a hemorrhagic complication to stroke. Since increasing availability of CT and MRI scans, lumbar puncture is only used infrequently due to the risk of brain stem herniation.

Ophthalmoscopy refers to the magnified visual inspection of the fundus of the eye. It may show signs of hypertension and atherosclerotic changes in the retinal arteries or evidence of cerebral edema.

Ocular plethysmiography measures blood flow through the tiny vessels in and around the eyes.

Electroencephalogram (EEG) consists of an electrical tracing of the brain waves that can localize the damaged area of the brain. It is usually used to document seizure activity, whether related to stroke or other neurological conditions.

Traditional Chinese Medicine & Stroke

In Chinese medicine, stroke is referred to as *zhong fen*, stroke [by] wind or wind stroke. As a disease entity, wind stroke has been recognized within the Chinese medical literature for at least 2,000 years. As mentioned above, the first extant description of various types of wind stroke are found in the *Nei Jing (Inner Classic)*, and, to this day, the fundamental theories of the causes and mechanisms of this class of disease mainly revolve around the concept of wind. In Chinese medicine, wind as a disease

cause may be either externally contracted or internally engendered. However, in general, it is said that, "prevalence of wind leads to stirring," as in tremors, and "prevalence of wind leads to drawing," as in contraction. In particular within Chinese medicine, wind evils are associated with hemiplegia and facial paralysis. Further, "The liver is the wind viscus." This means that internally engendered wind is primarily associated with the liver. Therefore, most cases of stroke involve some element of liver wind. In addition, most cases of stroke also involve some element of the Chinese medical concept of phlegm.

Disease causes and mechanisms

According to the theories of traditional Chinese medicine, stroke basically results from qi and blood counterflowing upward causing damage to the tissues of the brain. Internal wind is one of the most common disease mechanisms that results in stroke. However, there are many factors that can lead to this upward counterflow of qi and blood. These factors can be summarized into five main categories:

1. Age

Age is one of the leading factors predisposing one to stroke. As a person grows older, source or original qi decreases, resulting in an imbalance of yin and yang in the body. According to the *Nei Jing (Inner Classic)*, "[At] 40 years [of age], yin is automatically half." In particular, due to heart, liver, and kidney yin vacuity, yin may fail to control yang. Because "yin vacuity engenders internal heat" and "fire easily engenders wind," this may give rise, in turn, to the engenderment of internal stirring of liver wind. Because "blood and essence [share] a common source," it is also possible for a simple yin-blood vacuity to cause internal stirring of liver wind. In this case, "blood vacuity has no way to enclose the qi," and the qi counterflows chaotically upward in the form of wind.

2. Internal damage by the seven affects

Any greatly excessive affect or emotion may cause disease in its corresponding viscus. In particular, "explosive anger damages the liver" and "explosive anger damages yin." Thus explosive anger may lead to yin vacuity with internal heat and hence to the engenderment of liver wind. Therefore, it is said, "Extreme anger damaging the liver leads to dizziness and vertigo." However, it is also a statement of fact in Chinese medicine that, "Damage of the affects all lead to [diseases] pertaining to fire and heat." This means that excesses of any emotion, whether traditionally corresponding to the liver or not, may result in the engenderment of internal heat which further gives rise to stirring of liver wind. In addition,

> [If] a person is not able to achieve one's will [or desire], repression and depression damage the liver. [In that case,] liver wood is not able to course and discharge . . .

In other words, unfulfilled desires give rise to liver depression qi stagnation. If this depression is excessive or enduring, it may also transform internal heat which then may give rise to stirring of liver wind.

3. Unregulated food and drink

Alcohol and too much fatty, rich food can damage the spleen and impair its ability to transform and transport water fluids. If water fluids collect, they may transform into dampness, and, if dampness endures, it may congeal into phlegm. Therefore, the resulting spleen qi vacuity may engender phlegm. This is the reason it is traditionally said in Chinese medicine, "The spleen is the root of phlegm engenderment." However, once phlegm is engendered in the body, it hinders and obstructs the free flow of yang qi. The yang qi, which is inherently warm, becomes depressed and transforms into internally engendered heat. Because alcohol is hot in nature as well as damp-engendering, overconsumption of alcohol in particular is especially likely to give rise to heat in addition to phlegm. Once produced, this phlegm and heat typically combine together. In that case, the heat counterflows upward, commonly manifesting as wind, and drafts the phlegm along with it to the upper part of the body where it blocks and obstructs the clear orifices.

4. Externally contracted wind evils

Occasionally, external wind evils may invade the body. This occurs when the body is weak and deficient, as in the elderly. "The defensive qi exits from the middle burner" as the by-product of the process of digestion governed by the spleen. As we age, the spleen becomes vacuous and weak, and thus the defensive qi also commonly becomes insufficient. Such externally contracted wind evils lodge in the channels and vessels where they impede the free flow of the qi and blood, thus giving rise to symptoms of blockage and obstruction.

5. Constitution or body-type

While aging, emotional factors, improper diet, and external contraction of wind evils are the four main causes of stroke, we also must take into account the role of constitution in the occurrence of this disease. In Chinese medicine, it is believed that, due to our inheritance from our parents, each of us is predisposed to a certain body-type with varying amounts of qi and blood and yin and yang, and various strengths and weaknesses of the five viscera and six bowels. One body-type in particular is especially liable to the development of stroke, and this is called the *tai yang* or maximum yang body-type. This person has an inherent exuberance of yang qi. In other words, they have an exuberant ministerial/life-gate fire. When young, this yang qi exuberance led them to be strong and vigorous with a large appetite. However, as these individuals age, their spleen becomes vacuous and weak like the rest of us, while their stomach remains relatively hot and replete. This means these people continue to eat a lot and often to eat a lot of rich, fatty foods which they previously were able to digest without gaining weight. But now, because of the weakening of the spleen, they are not able to transform and transport the essence and fluids of these foods. Instead, these pathologically transform into phlegm, dampness, and turbidity and so they gain weight. Because of the especially close relationship of the ministerial/life-gate fire with the liver, gallbladder, and stomach, these patients also typically have a hot or yang exuberant liver. As it is said, "The life-gate, triple burner, and ministerial fire all attach to [or connect with] the liver-gallbladder." Therefore, these persons are especially prone to developing phlegm heat which may further engender liver wind.

As for what this body-type looks like, the *tai yang* person has an overdeveloped upper body and underdeveloped lower body. They have a large chest with strong muscles above but often thin buttocks and legs. Their face tends to be red and they suffer with age from central obesity or a so-called beer-belly. They may be either male or female, but more often than not are male. They also tend to be easily excitable and even angry. We all know and have seen

people with this *tai yang* body-type, and it is these people who should be especially careful about their emotions and diet. These people should eat less fatty, rich food and drink less alcohol. Instead, they should eat more vegetables, fruits, and whole grains. They should try to lose weight, and they should try to relax and not be angry.

The Chinese medical classification of strokes

In Chinese medicine, stroke or wind stroke is not a single entity. Just as Western medicine identifies five different nosologies of stroke manifestations, Chinese medicine also divides stroke into two main and four subcategories. This system of classification was originally described in the Zhang Zhong-jing's *Jin Gui Yao Lue (Essentials of the Golden Cabinet)* in the early 3rd century or Eastern Han dynasty but is still widely used in clinical practice today.

In stroke of the **network vessels** (*zhong luo*), wind attacks the network vessels. There is numbness of the skin and deviation of the eye and mouth on one side of the face. This is the very mildest type of stroke in Chinese medicine.

Stroke of the **channels** (*zhong jing*) is more serious, just as the channels are larger and more important than the network vessels. In this case, there is paralysis of an arm and a leg (hemiplegia). Dysphagia and aphasia may also occur.

In stroke of the **bowels** (*zhong fu*), the patient may suddenly lose consciousness. Upon awakening, the patient may be hemiplegic and/or incontinent or exhibit symptoms such as the retention of urine and constipation. In Chinese medicine, these are considered "tense" symptoms, and the two

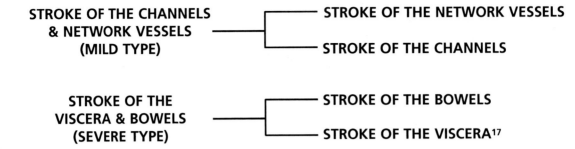

types of stroke of the viscera and bowels are differentiated by the presence of tense or flaccid symptoms.

In stroke of the **viscera** (*zhong zang*), the patient is unconscious and comatose with open mouth, drooping lips, and dribbling saliva. These are all flaccid symptoms, and this is the most severe type of stroke.

The sequelae of stroke

After the stroke patient has been stabilized, there may be enduring paralysis on one side of the body or hemiplegia. The patient may have motor impairment of the arm and/or leg and the muscles may be either flaccid or spastic. Persistent spasticity may lead to contractures across joints. For the most part, it is these sequelae which we practitioners of acupuncture are called on to treat. When these sequelae are mostly associated with flaccidity of the muscles, the condition falls under the Chinese medical category of wilting condition (*wei zheng*). When they are associated with spasticity, they typically fall under the general Chinese medical category of hypertonicity of the four limbs (*si zhi ji ju*). In addition, specific symptoms fall under other individual Chinese medical disease categories. For instance, there are tremors of the hands (*shou chan*), tremors of the feet (*zu chan*), tremor of the head (*tou yao*), deviated mouth and eye (*kou yan wai xie*), numbness of the face (*yan mian*

ma mu), drooling from the corner of the mouth (*kou jiao liu xian*), and stiff tongue (*she qiang*). For more information on the disease mechanisms, pattern discrimination, and Chinese medical treatment of these specific disease categories, please see Philippe Sionneau and Lu Gang's¸ *The Treatment of Disease in TCM* also available from Blue Poppy Press.

Endnotes

[1] Yu Zhi-shun, *et al.*, *Zhong Guo Zhen Jiu Za Zhi (Journal of Chinese Acupuncture & Moxibustion)*, 1985, #4, p. 21-24

[2] American Heart Association, "Heart Disease and Stroke Statistics," *http://www.american heart.org* in 2004

[3] "Stroke Fact Sheet," Centers for Disease Control, this document came from their website in 1997, and can be accessed at: *http://www.cdc.gov*

[4] *Ibid.*

[5] R. F. Macko, *et al.*, "Treadmill Aerobic Exercise Training Reduces the Energy Expenditure and Cardiovascular Demands of Hemi paretic Gait in Chronic Stroke Patients— A Preliminary Report," *Stroke*, American Heart Association, 1997, Vol. 28, #2, p. 326-330

[6] L. Wolfson, "Gait and Balance Dysfunction: A Model of the Interaction of Age and Disease," *Neuroscientist*, 2001, #2, p.178-183

[7] S. F. Farmer *et al.*, "Change in Motor Unit Synchronization Following Central Nervous Lesions in Man, *Journal of Physiology,* 463, p. 83-105

[8] Oscar Foder, M.D., "Epidemiology of

Stroke," presented his speech at the symposium Current Advances in Stroke, Seattle, WA, U.S.A. on June 19, 1986

[9] Information was given by Zheng Ban-tsan, former Chief Director of Acupuncture Department of Chongqing Research Institute of Traditional Chinese Medicine, Chongqing, China, 1984

[10] Foder, *op. cit.*

[11] American Heart Association, "News," March 18, 1988, Santa Fe, United Press International

[12] Robert C. Goiney, M.D., "Diagnostic Imaging in Diagnosis of Stroke," presented his speech at the symposium Current Advances in Stroke, Seattle, WA, U.S.A. on June 19, 1986

[13] Foder, *op. cit.*

[14] Foder, *op. cit.*

[15] Simeon Margolis, M.D., Ph.D. & Robert J. Wityk, M.D., "Stroke," *The Johns Hopkins White Papers,* Baltimore, MD, U.S.A., 1998, p. 5

[16] *Ibid.*, p. 8

[17] *Ibid.*, p. 26

[18] *Jian Ming Zhong Yi Ci Dian, (A Concise Chinese Medical Dictionary)*, People's Health Publishing, Beijing, 1979, p. 135 & p. 532

TWO
Review of Standard Acupuncture Therapy for Stroke and Its Rehabilitation

Before immediately looking at the many published contemporary reports of clinical trials on the use of acupuncture in the treatment of stroke, I (HPYC) believe it is useful to briefly review the textbook or school approach to this subject. Acupuncture is an ancient healing art that has been practiced for thousands of years, and throughout this long history of Chinese medicine, many experienced physicians have recorded their valuable clinical experiences regarding stroke. These experiences may be found in numerous classical and premodern acupuncture texts. In addition, certain treatments have become standard in China today. Therefore, when it comes to the textbook treatments of stroke, we can divide these into classical, standard first-aid, and standard rehabilitative therapies for the acupuncture treatment of stroke and its sequelae. The classical treatments reviewed below are for the immediate relief of the acute symptoms of stroke and for resuscitation and are taken from some of the most important premodern Chinese medical texts. The standard first aid treatments presented below are also for the immediate relief of the acute symptoms of stroke and reflect standard contemporary practice in China.

As the reader will see, even in contemporary clinical practice, practitioners base first aid treatment on whether the patient manifests a tense or flaccid presentation. And finally, the standard rehabilitative treatments included herein are for the treatment of the sequelae of stroke after the patient has been stabilized. These are standard or textbook treatments in the People's Republic of China as well and are also commonly taught at Western acupuncture schools and colleges.

Classical Treatments for Stroke

Tense symptoms

The patient is in an acute condition, going in and out of consciousness, with a deep red facial complexion. His or her mouth and hands are tightly closed with generalized muscular clenching. The patient's breathing is heavy with the sound of sputum. He or she is unable to urinate or defecate and has a bowstring[1], slippery, and fast pulse.

According to Sun Si-miao in the Tang dynasty in his *Qian Jin Yi Fang*

(Supplement to Prescriptions Worth A Thousand [Pieces of] Gold):

> For clenched jaws, use *Jia Che* (St 6) with moxibustion, five cones bilaterally.

> For unconscious, use *Ren Zhong* (GV 26). Use draining technique applied with a needle.

According to Yang Ji-zhou in the Ming dynasty in his *Zhen Jiu Da Cheng (Compendium of Acupuncture & Moxibustion)*:

> For clenched jaws, use *Jia Che* (St 6), *Ren Zhong* (GV 26), *He Gu* (LI 4), *Bai Hui* (GV 20), and *Cheng Jiang* (CV 24). Use draining technique with needles on all these points. If there is still no response, then use *Lian Quan* (CV 23).

> For unconscious, use *Ren Zhong* (GV 26), *Zhong Chong* (Per 9), *He Gu* (LI 4), and *Ya Men* (GV 15). If there is no response, add *Da Dun* (Liv 1).

Flaccid symptoms

Patient is in collapse due to an acute yang vacuity condition with a pale facial complexion and tightly closed eyes but an open mouth. In addition, there is sweating, cold and extended limbs, uncontrolled elimination, prostration, and breathing with snore.

According to the *Qian Jin Yi Fang*:

> Moxa *Bai Hui* (GV 20) with 700 cones.

According to Zhang Jie-bin (a.k.a. Zhang Jing-yue) in his Ming dynasty *Lei Jing (The Systematized [Inner] Classic)*:

Use moxibustion with salt and ginger on *Shen Que* (GV 8) with 100-500 cones.

Standard First Aid Treatments

Tense symptoms

Treatment principles: Clear heat and arouse the spirit (i.e., resuscitate), downbear counterflow

Treatment method: This protocol uses three groups of points.

1. Regulate the qi of the governing vessel and effect resuscitation by needling *Bai Hui* (GV 20) and *Ren Zhong* (GV 26) with strong stimulation.

2. Bleed the 12 well points to clear heat in the upper part of the body, thus causing the internal wind to subside. These 12 points are *Shao Shang* (Lu 11), *Shang Yang* (LI 1), *Zhong Chong* (Per 9), *Guan Chong* (TB 1), *Shao Chong* (Ht 9), and *Shao Ze* (SI 1).

3. Lead heat to move downward using *Yong Quan* (Ki 1). This is based on the method of choosing points below to treat a disease above.

Auxiliary points include *Nei Guan* (Per 6) and *Lao Gong* (Per 8) for calming the heart and quieting the spirit. *Feng Chi* (GB 20) for dispelling the wind and clearing the mind, and bleeding the *Shi Xuan* (M-UE-1) to drain counterflowing blood.

Flaccid symptoms

Treatment principles: Rescue yang and stem desertion

Treatment method: This protocol uses four sets of points.

1. As first aid to restore the vital functions of the conception vessel, moxa *Guan Yuan* (CV 4), *Qi Hai* (CV 6), and *Shen Que* (CV 8) indirectly over salt and ginger.

2. To free the flow of the qi mechanism, use *Zu San Li* (St 36) and *Da Dun* (Liv 1).

3. To arouse the spirit and restore consciousness, needle *Ren Zhong* (GV 26) and moxa *Bai Hui* (GV 20).

4. For supplementing the exhausted source or original qi, use *Shan Zhong* (CV 17), *Shen Shu* (Bl 23), and *Ming Men* (GV 4). Use supplementation or mild stimulation with continuous application of moxibustion to the points on the conception and governing vessels.[2]

Standard Acupuncture Treatments for the Various Sequelae of Stroke

Treatment principles: Free the flow of the channels and open the network vessels, dispel wind and quicken the blood

Treatment method:

For general regulation of the qi in the body, use *Bai Hui* (GV 20), *Tong Tian* (Bl 7), and *Feng Fu* (GV16).

Wind, being a yang evil, usually affects the upper and exterior parts of the body. *Feng Fu, Bai Hui,* and *Tong Tian* are, therefore, used to dispel wind. Because the yang channels govern the exterior of the body, points are chosen mainly on the yang channels to regulate and rectify the qi and blood of the body and promote smooth circulation in the channels and network vessels.

For paralysis of the arm, needle *He Gu* (LI 4), *Zhong Zhu* (TB 3), *Qu Chi* (LI 11), *Wai Guan* (TB 5), *Jian Yu* (LI 15), and *Jian Liao* (TB 14) on the affected side.

The *yang ming* channels have lots of qi and lots of blood. Therefore, points on the large intestine channel are selected first, while points on the triple burner channel are used adjunctively.

For paralysis of the leg, needle *Fu Tu* (St 32), *Huan Tiao* (GB 30), *Zu San Li* (St 36), *Feng Chi* (GB 31), *Jie Xi* (St 41), and *Yang Ling Quan* (GB 34) on the affected side.

For the same reason, the points on the stomach channel are the primary ones in the above formula, while the points on the gallbladder channel are adjunctive.

For facial paralysis, needle *Si Bai* (St 2), *Xia Guan* (St 7), *Di Cang* (St 4), *Yi Feng* (TB 17), *Jia Che* (St 6), and *He Gu* (LI 4) on the affected side.

In this case, even supplementing-even draining treatment is used on points on the *yang ming* to dispel wind and free the flow of the network vessels. In addition, both the hand and foot *yang ming* channels transverse the cheek.[3]

For clenched jaws, use *Jia Che* (St 6), *Xia Guan* (St 7), and He Gu (LI 4).

These points on the *yang ming* channels are chosen for the same reasons as for facial paralysis above.

For gurgling with sputum, use *Tian Tu* (CV 22), *Feng Long* (St 40), and *Nei Guan* (Per 6) to course the qi and transform phlegm.

For aphasia and stiffness of the tongue, use *Ya Men* (GV 15), *Lian Quan* (CV 23), and *Tong Li* (Ht 5).

In this case, *Ya Men* and *Lian Quan* are local points which free the flow of the channel qi. *Tong Li* is the network point of the heart channel. This point is used to resolve stiffness of the tongue because the tongue is the sprout of the heart.

For urinary incontinence, moxa *Guan Yuan* (CV 4) and *Zhong Ji* (CV 3) and needle *San Yin Jiao* (Sp 6), and *Tai Xi* (Ki 3) with supplementing technique in order to supplement the kidney qi.

For symptoms associated with fire, such as a flushed face, thirst, irritability, and constipation, needle *Da Ling* (Per 7), the stream and source point of the pericardium channel, *Xing Jian* (Liv 2), the fire point of the liver channel, *Tian Shu* (St 25), the *mu* or alarm point of the large intestine, and *Shang Ju Xu* (St 37), the lower uniting point of the large intestine which is indicated for disorders of the large intestine such as constipation.

For symptoms associated with ascension of liver wind, such as convulsions, headache, dizziness, and spasms of the hands and feet, use *Tai Chong* (Liv 3), the stream and source point of the liver channel which directly treats the offending viscus, and *Yang Ling Quan* (GB 34), the uniting point of the gallbladder which clears heat in the liver-gallbladder.[4]

Endnotes

[1] Wiseman & Feng's term is stringlike. Many practitioners use the term wiry. However, the Chinese character clearly shows a drawn bowstring. Wiseman, Nigel & Feng Ye, *A Practical Dictionary of Chinese Medicine*, Paradigm Publications, Brookline, MA, 1999, p. 584

[2] Beijing College of Traditional Chinese Medicine *et al.*, *Essentials of Chinese Acupuncture*, Foreign Languages Press, Beijing, 1980, p. 332-335

[3] Shanghai College of Traditional Chinese Medicine, *Zhen Jiu Xue (A Study of Acupuncture & Moxibustion)* published in English under the title, *Acupuncture: A Comprehensive Text,* edited and translated by John O'Connor and Dan Bensky, Eastland Press, Chicago, 1981, p. 619-620

[4] Tian Cong-hua, *A Collection of Acupuncture & Moxibustion Medical Experiences*, Science & Technology Articles Publishing Company, Chongqing, China, 1985, p. 521

THREE
Experiences in the Treatment of Stroke from Recognized Experts in the Field

As this book amply demonstrates, there are a variety of ways to approach the treatment of stroke with acupuncture. In this chapter, we present the techniques of a group of especially well-known and respected Chinese acupuncturists for the treatment of various symptoms related to stroke.

Wang Le-ting's 13 Treatment Methods for Stroke[1]

Wang Le-ting was a famous Chinese doctor in Beijing and had more than 50 years experience in treating stroke patients. His treatments were so effective that people called him "Golden Needle Wang". Practitioners can choose from the following 13 protocols depending on which might be most beneficial for each individual patient at the time of treatment. When there is more than a single protocol for the same purpose, Dr. Wang would often use one protocol for a week at a time, alternating or cycling through the protocols week by week. In general, Dr. Wang treated daily or every other day depending on the severity of the condition.

1. Protocol for tense symptoms

This formula is for resuscitation and bring-ing one back to consciousness from coma. It has two steps.

First, the following points are each pricked to bleed 1-3 drops: *Bai Hui* (GV 20), *Si Shen Cong* (M-HN-1), and the 12 well points.

Secondly, the following points are nee-dled with draining technique: *Ren Zhong* (GV 26), *Cheng Jiang* (CV 24), *Feng Chi* (GB 20), *Feng Fu* (GV 16), *He Gu* (LI 4), *Lao Gong* (Per 8), *Tai Chong* (Liv 3), and *Yong Quan* (Ki 1)

2. Protocol for flaccid symptoms

This formula is meant to restore yang and stem desertion and as an emergency treat-ment for prostration. It has three steps.

Step one, moxa *Shen Que* (CV 8) indi-rectly with roasted salt and a slice of ginger placed on top of the salt. Up to 100 large moxa cones can be burned.

Step two, use direct moxibustion on *Qi Hai* (CV 6) and *Guan Yuan* (CV 4), burn-ing up to 100 small cones or until a pulse is felt and the limbs become warm again.

Step three, use supplementation technique on *Bai Hui* (GV 20), *Zu San Li* (St 36), *Nei Guan* (Per 6), and *Yong Quan* (Ki 1).

3. Protocol for hemiplegia

The following was the main formula Dr. Wang used for hemiplegia. It is called 12 Needles on the Arms and Legs. It consists of three points on the arms and another three points on the legs all needled bilaterally, thus giving a total of 12 needles. The three points on the arms are *Qu Chi* (LI 11), *He Gu* (LI 4), and *Nei Guan* (Per 6). The three points on the legs are *Zu San Li* (St 36), *Yang Ling Quan* (GB 34), and *San Yin Jiao* (Sp 6).

4. An alternate protocol for hemiplegia

This protocol uses 14 needles all on the paralyzed side: *Bai Hui* (GV 20), *Feng Fu* (GV 16), *Feng Chi* (GB 20), *Jian Jing* (GB 21), *Jian Yu* (LI 15), *Qu Chi* (LI 11), *He Gu* (LI 4), *Lei Que* (Lu 7), *Huan Tiao* (GB 30), *Wei Zhong* (Bl 40), *Yang Ling Quan* (GB 34), *Xuan Zhong* (GB 39), *Qiu Xu* (GB 40), and *Tai Chong* (Liv 3)

5. Protocol for long-term, rigid type hemiplegia

Dr. Wang used this protocol for the symptoms of inability to raise the shoulder, spastic elbow, dropped wrist, clenched fist, rigid hip, knee, and/or ankle, inversion and eversion of the foot, walking with a limp, and inability to lift up the foot. It employs the acupuncture technique called point joining. This entails using a single needle to penetrate through from one point to another. Dr. Wang's stated purpose for using this technique was to achieve stronger stimulation. Dr. Wang's 12 joined

needles formula consists of: (*Arrows mean needled through to*)

Feng Chi (GB 20) ⟶ *Feng Fu* (GV 16)
Jian Yu (LI 15) ⟶ *Bi Nao* (LI 14)
Qu Chi (LI 11) ⟶ *Shao Hai* (Ht 3)
Wai Guan (TB 5) ⟶ *Nei Guan* (Per 6)
Yang Chi (TB 4) ⟶ *Da Ling* (Per 7)
He Gu (LI 4) ⟶ *Lao Gong* (Per 8)
Huan Tiao (GB 30) ⟶ *Feng Shi* (GB 31)
Xi Yang Guan (GB 33) ⟶ *Qu Quan* (Liv 8)
Yang Ling Quan (GB 34) > *Yin Ling Quan* (Sp 9)
Xuan Zhong (GB 39) ⟶ *San Yin Jiao* (Sp 6)
Ku Lun (Bl 60) ⟶ *Tai Xi* (Ki 3)
Tai Chong (Liv 3) ⟶ *Yong Quan* (Ki 1)

6. Protocol for facial paralysis

This formula employs eight needles, all on the face. The points consist of *Ren Zhong* (GV 26), *Cheng Jiang* (CV 24), *Si Bai* (St 2), *Di Cang* (St 40), *Da Ying* (St 5), *Jia Che* (St 6), *Quan Liao* (SI 18), and *Yang Bai* (GB 14) needled on the affected side.

7. Protocol for severe, long-term facial paralysis

This formula uses eight pairs of joined needles to achieve greater stimulation in moving the qi and freeing the flow of the channels:

Yang Bai (GB 14) ⟶ *Yu Yao* (M-HN-6)
Zan Zhu (Bl 2) ⟶ *Si Zhu Kong* (TB 23)
Si Bai (St 2) ⟶ *Cheng Qi* (St 1)
Feng Chi (GB 20) ⟶ *Feng Fu* (GV 16)
Tai Yang (M-HN-9) ⟶ *Quan Liao* (SI 18)
He Liao (LI 19) ⟶ *Ju Liao* (St 3)
Di Cang (St 4) ⟶ *Jia Che* (St 6)

These points are needled on the affected side. In addition, *Qu Chi* (LI 11) and *He Gu* (LI 4) are needled on the affected side since the hand *yang ming* traverses the side of the face.

8. Protocol for yang vacuity to upbear the clear

Dr. Wang called this formula 13 Needles on the Governing Vessel:

Bai Hui (GV 20), *Feng Fu* (GV 16), *Da Zhui* (GV 14), *Tao Dao* (GV 13), *Shen Zhu* (GV 12), *Shen Dao* (GV 11), *Zhi Yang* (GV 9), *Jin Suo* (GV 8), *Ji Zhong* (GV 6), *Xuan Shu* (GV 5), *Ming Men* (GV 4), *Yao Yang Quan* (GV 3), and *Chang Qiang* (GV 1)

The governing vessel is the sea of yang among the channels and vessels and the head is the reunion of yang. Consciousness, the ability to think, and functions of the eyes, ears, and mouth are all expressions of the clear yang which, at least in part, is upborne to the head by the governing vessel.

9. Protocol for directing yin to yang as well as regulating the qi in the *chong mai* and conception vessel

Dr. Wang called this formula 12 Needles on the Conception Vessel. It consists of *Cheng Jiang* (CV 24), *Lian Quan* (CV 23), *Tian Tu* (CV 22), *Zi Gong* (CV 19), *Shan Zhong* (CV 17), *Jiu Wei* (CV 15), *Shang Wan* (CV 13), *Zhong Wan* (CV 12), *Xia Wan* (CV 10), *Qi Hai* (CV 6), *Guan Yuan* (CV 4), and *Zhong Ji* (CV 3), plus moxibustion on *Shen Que* (CV 8). The governing and conception vessels run into and connect with each other. As stated above, it was a principle of Dr. Wang's not to repeat a single formula too many times, thus desensitizing the points. It was also a principle of his that, if he was needling on the front of the body, he only needled on the front, and if he was needling on the back, he only needled on the back. This was because he was such a busy clinician and did not have the time to turn patients over from side to side. Thus he developed ways of accomplishing what he

wanted to do all from one side or the other.

10. Protocol for vacuity of the five viscera

This next formula Dr. Wang called the Five Transports Plus *Ge Shu*. He used it to supplement the source qi of the five viscera. After long-term hemiplegia, typically the qi, blood, yin, and yang all become vacuous and weak. In addition, needling the back transport points of the lungs, heart, liver, spleen, and kidneys harmonizes the functions of these five organs. Dr. Wang's formula consists of *Fei Shu* (Bl 13), *Xin Shu* (Bl 15), *Ge Shu* (Bl 17), *Gan Shu* (Bl 18), *Pi Shu* (Bl 20), and *Shen Shu* (Bl 23).

11. Protocol for freeing the flow of the six bowels

Likewise, after long-term hemiplegia, symptoms of stagnation of six bowels tend to appear, such as constipation and urinary retention. Needling the back transport points of the gallbladder, stomach, triple burner, large intestine, small intestine, and urinary bladder harmonizes and frees the flow of these six bowels. Dr. Wang's formula consists of *Dan Shu* (Bl 19), *Wei Shu* (Bl 21), *San Jiao Shu* (Bl 22), *Da Chang Shu* (Bl 25), *Xiao Chang Shu* (Bl 27), and *Pang Guan Shu* (Bl 28). These points can all be needled at once or several of them pertaining to a particular symptom might be chosen, for instance, *Wei Shu*, *Da Chang Shu*, and *Xiao Chang Shu* for constipation or *San Jiao Shu*, *Xiao Chang Shu*, and *Pang Guan Shu* for urinary retention. In other words, Dr. Wang meant these formulas to be used flexibly.

12. Protocol for dysfunction of the viscera and bowels

Dr. Wang also used the nine front *mu* or

alarm points corresponding to their associated viscera and bowels. It should be remembered that both the back transport and front *mu* points have a direct connection to their associated viscera and bowels unmediated by the channels and vessels. That makes these points especially powerful for stimulating their corresponding organs. Dr. Wang's formula consists of *Zhong Fu* (Lu 1), *Shan Zhong* (CV17), *Ju Que* (CV 14), *Qi Men* (Liv 14), *Zhang Men* (Liv 13), *Zhong Wan* (CV 12), *Tian Shu* (St 25), *Guan Yuan* (CV 4), and *Zhong Ji* (CV 3). Again, these points may be used altogether at one time or in selective combinations depending on the patient's symptoms.

13. Protocol for dysfunction of the digestive system

This formula is one of Wang Le-ting's most famous. It is called Old Ten Needles and is for any patient suffering the symptoms of disharmony of the spleen and stomach, including loss of appetite, indigestion, abdominal distention, belching and hiccup. The formula consists of *Shang Wan* (CV 13), *Zhong Wan* (CV 12), *Xia Wan* (CV 10), *Qi Hai* (CV 6), *Nei Guan* (Per 6), *Tian Shu* (St 25), and *Zu San Li* (St 36).

The combination of *Shang Wan*, *Zhong Wan*, and *Xia Wan* is called the three ducts and strongly disinhibits the qi mechanism. Old Ten Needles is mostly for digestive complaints stemming from stagnation and repletion of the stomach and intestines. If there is more pronounced spleen qi vacuity, then *Shang Wan* and *Xia Wan* are replaced by *Zhang Men* (Liv 13) and the formula is then called Old Replete Needles.

As a general rule, for acute cases, Dr. Wang emphasized treating the symptoms (*i.e.*, the so-called tips or branches). Then, after the emergency condition was stabilized, he emphasized treating the original source or root. Dr. Wang especially emphasized that treatment should be based on the health condition of the individual's whole body as shown by the different presenting symptoms. For more information on Dr. Wang's theories, needle techniques, and formulas, see *Golden Needle Wang Le-ting* also available from Blue Poppy Press.

Jiao Shun-fa's Scalp Needling Method[2]

Scalp needling is a special acupuncture technique which was developed from a combination of Chinese medical theory and neuro-anatomical physiology. This technique is especially good for the treatment of brain diseases or symptoms related to the cerebral cortex. It entails needling the scalp at points corresponding to functional areas of the cerebral cortex. In other words, the areas stimulated by this therapy are primarily determined by the localization of the associated cerebral cortical function projected onto the scalp. This technique was invented and developed by Jiao Shun-fa. Prof. Jiao began his research on scalp acupuncture in 1965 and successfully applied it for paralysis caused by central nervous system dysfunction. This technique has proven itself so effective that, by 1971, the study and practice of scalp needling became nationally accepted in China.

The "points" used in this system are actually lines or zones. In general, when using this technique for the treatment of unilateral sequelae of stroke, one chooses points on the scalp opposite to the affected side. When the symptoms are bilateral, points on both hemispheres of the scalp are used. Typically, 26-28 gauge, 2.5-3 inch fine needles are inserted subcutaneously in a particular direction along one or more of these lines. The needles are inserted in a twisting manner to the proper depth. Lifting or pushing of the needle is not necessary. After the needle is in the proper place, the needle is twisted at the frequency of approximately 200 times per minute. Generally, after 30 seconds to one minute of stimulation, the corresponding limb will feel warm, numb, distended, and/or sore. The practitioner then continues twisting the needle for 3-5 minutes. Then he or she lets the needle rest in place for 5-10 minutes. The needles are withdrawn after repeating the above stimulation 2-3 times. When doing scalp needling, strict sterilization is required to avoid any infection. Below are summaries of three articles on clinical trials in which authors used Jiao's scalp needling technique for the treatment of stroke patients.

The first article describes the treatment of 444 cases of paralysis and aphasia due to stroke.[3] In this study the main scalp needling zone employed was the so-called motor area. Auxiliary zones or lines included the foot motor and sensory areas. If there was numbness in the limbs, then the sensory area was also needled. If there was edema in the limbs or hypertension, blood vessel dilation and constriction areas were added. If there was aphasia, speech area I was added for motor aphasia and speech area III was added for sensory aphasia. Twenty-six to 28 gauge, 40-50mm needles were inserted at an angle of 30 degrees into the indicated areas or zones. The needles were then connected to an electro-acupuncture machine with a frequency of 130-400 cycles per minute. The electric current was left on for approximately two minutes. Then needles were retained for 20 minutes. Patients were treated per day or once every other day, and 15 treatments equaled one

course. In the first group of 335 cases with cerebral paralysis, 208 cases (62.1%) were cured, 58 cases (17.3%) obtained a marked effect, and another 49 cases (14.6%) improved. Only 20 cases (6%) got no effect. Therefore, the total effectiveness rate in this group was 94%. In the second group of 109 cases of aphasia, 67 cases (61.5%) were cured, 19 cases (17.4%) got a marked effect, and 15 cases (13.8%) improved. Only eight of these cases (7.3%) got no effect, for a total effectiveness rate of 92.7%. It was the belief of the authors of this study that improvement of the circulation of blood in the damaged portions of the cerebral cortex is the main reason for the success of this technique in stroke victims.

The second article describes the treatment of 24 cases of hemiplegia with scalp acupuncture.[4] Among these 24 cases, there were 13 males and 11 females 43-87 years of age with an average age of 59.3 years. Eighteen of these cases had been given cephalic CT scans and all diagnoses matched the criteria for hemiplegia due to stroke set by the Second National Academic Meeting of Neuropsychiatry. The selection of scalp acupoints was based on the corresponding functional areas according to the division of the cerebral cortex. Motor and sensory zones on the opposite side of the hemiplegic limbs were chosen. Speech area I was needled in the case of aphasia. Electrical stimulation was applied to all points using a frequency of 120-140 cycles per minute. The strength of this stimulation was as great as each individual could bear. Treatment was given once daily for 30 minutes. Patients had six treatments per week followed by one day of rest. Three weeks of treatment equaled one course. At the end of the study, seven cases (29.2%) got a marked effect, 13 cases (54.1%) got some effect, and four cases (16.6%) got no effect.

Therefore, the total effectiveness rate was 83.3%). In addition, the results of this study showed that the shorter the time after the occurrence of the stroke, the better the therapeutic effects.

The third article describes an even larger cohort of patients treated for hemiplegia by scalp needling on the motor, sensory, and speech areas on the side opposite the afflicted limbs.[5] In some of the complicated cases, needles were also added on other scalp areas. Further, the authors used three different kinds of manipulation to compare their relative effects. In group I, manual rotation of the needles was used every 3-5 minutes at a rate of 200-250 twists per minute. This was performed a total of three times. Then needles were retained for 15 minutes. Treatment was given once per day, with 20 treatments equaling one course.[6] In group II, an electrical rotating device twisted the needles at a speed of 300 times per minute. The needles were retained for 15 minutes, treatment was given once daily, and 20 treatments also equaled one course. In group III, the needles were connected to a G 6805 electro-acupuncture device. Continuous waves were used at a frequency of 500-700 cycles per minute. After 10 minutes of stimulation, the needles were retained for another 15 minutes. Frequency and course of treatment were the same as above. All patients in the three groups took a 5-7 day break after each course before resuming the next course. In group I, 104 out of 218 cases were cured, for a cure rate of 47.3%. In group II, 109 cases out of 216 were cured, for a cure rate of 50.46%, and, in group III, 395 cases out of 794 were cured, for a cure rate of 49.62%. Therefore, there was no statistically significant difference between the three groups in terms of

their rate of cure. The total effectiveness rate of 1228 cases was 98.53%.

Jiao's scalp acupuncture has been widely used by acupuncturists in China for over 30 years. During that time, it has proven to be a very effective technique for treating stroke conditions. Also during that time, many different scalp needling techniques have been developed, and there are many reports and articles discussing their remarkable results in treating stroke in the Chinese medical literature. I believe that, no matter what kind of scalp needling technique is used, we have to give credit to its inventor, Dr. Jiao Shun-fa and his Scalp Acupuncture Research Group in Yun Cheng District Hospital of Shanxi Province, China.

Zhu Ming-qing's Scalp Needling Technique[7]

I was fortunate enough to attend the First World Conference of Acupuncture-Moxibustion held by the World Federation of Acupuncture and Moxibustion Societies in Beijing on November 22-26, 1987. It was truly a learning experience that allowed me to share my knowledge with other

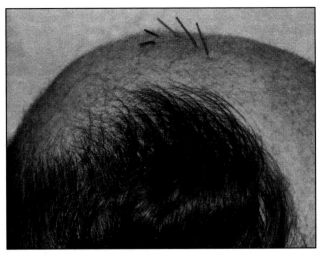

Zhu's scalp needles inserted on a patient's head.

acupuncturists from around the world. I was deeply impressed by the scalp needling technique demonstrated by Dr. Zhu Mingqing (now known as Mingqing Zhu in the U.S.) for the treatment of stroke patients. During the conference, Dr. Zhu demonstrated his special technique in front of more than 1,000 delegates. He treated two stroke patients by using scalp acuzones. These two patients were in wheelchairs, and they seemed very nervous. Dr. Zhu had never seen either of them before. The first patient had not received any acupuncture since suffering his stroke four months previously. He could not walk or stand. Dr. Zhu used his skillful and smooth technique to insert four needles on the following scalp acupuncture zones:

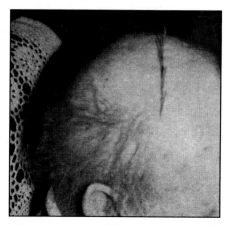

Another example of Zhu's scalp needling.

Zone 1: Anterior 1/4 of *E Ding* zone is at *Shen Ting* (GV 24) area to calm the mind
Zone 1: Posterior 1/4 of *E Ding* zone is at *Qian Ding* (GV 21) area to supplement kidney qi
Zone 6: *Ding Nie* zone is 0.5 inches anterior and posterior from the line from *Qian Ding* (GV 21) to *Tou Wei* (St 8) area

He inserted two needles on the side opposite of the paralyzed limbs in order to course the channels and strengthen the sinews. While he was manipulating the needles, his assistant was kneeling on the floor helping to move the patient's paralyzed legs. After manipulating for approximately 10 minutes, Dr. Zhu asked the patient to stand up. The patient was somewhat shaky at first but improved after some encouragement. Dr. Zhu then asked the patient to walk back and forth around the stage with the needles still in his scalp. He did this with some amazement. The second patient was then treated in a like manner. Both patients had been unable to stand or walk prior to the treatments. After 10 minutes of treatment, both

were able to stand and walk around the stage unassisted. All the delegates responded enthusiastically to the demonstration and obvious success of the treatments.

For the purpose of learning more about this technique, I asked Dr. Zhu to personally share more information with me about his treatment methods. He explained that, in his more than 20 years of clinical experience in treating stroke patients, the head acupoints produced the most effective results. Dr. Zhu summarized his experience as follows:

1. His favorite choice when performing scalp acupuncture for hemiplegia is the four acuzones on the head that were used in his demonstration.

2. He uses the manipulation technique known as the *chou qi* (whip the qi) method which uses very strong draining stimulation to the scalp area.

3. His treatment method combines the use of acupuncture with passive mobilization of the paralyzed limbs. According to Dr. Zhu, this is extremely important for achieving quick results.

4. He stresses that the practitioner needs

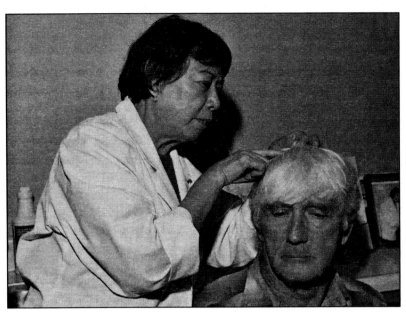

Dr. Chan using scalp acupuncture on one of her patients.

stroke and other paralytic patients with satisfactory results.

Peng Jinshan's Periocular Needling Method[8]

Periocular acupuncture was developed by Prof. Peng Jinshan who had practiced acupuncture and Chinese medicine for more than 60 years. He was famous in both China and around the world. Prof. Peng had continuously studied and practiced ocular diagnosis and periocular acupuncture techniques since 1970. The discovery of these techniques has been recognized by the Chinese government as a significant event in the growth of acupuncture science.

a lot of practice with this special manipulating technique. It is not as simple as it may appear and cannot be mastered overnight.

Dr. Zhu was invited to come to Seattle by the Northwest Institute of Acupuncture and Oriental Medicine in 1989 to teach his scalp needling technique and to share his expertise with more acupuncturists. He currently resides and practices in California. Since I have learned this special scalp needle technique, I use it in my practice for

According to Prof. Peng, periocular acupuncture for treating stroke is based on the theory of channels and network vessels taught by Hua Tou. Inspired by this unique technique, I made a special trip in 1993 to the Liaoning College of Chinese Medicine to do advanced study of this technique at his Ocular Acupuncture Research Department. The results of this technique deeply impressed me.

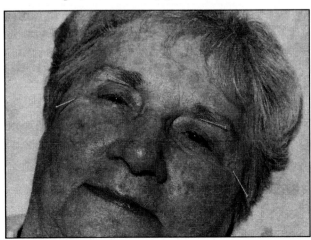

Periocular acupuncture zones location[14]

With the patient's eyes looking straight ahead, draw an imaginary

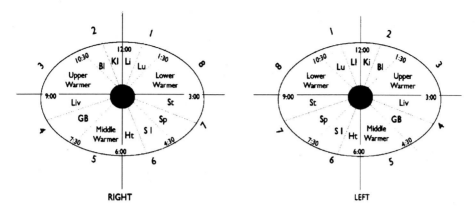

The Location of Ocular and Periocular Acupuncture Zones [9] (Triple Warmer is the same as Triple Burner)

horizontal line from the inner canthus through the center of the pupil to the outer canthus. Draw a second line vertically intersecting through the center of the pupil and eye. This divides the eye into four quadrants. Next, divide each quadrant in half creating the eight equal regions that are associated with 13 organs. Five of these regions are divided again into two equal zones. The other three regions that are not divided are the three burners which each occupy one zone as upper, middle and lower burner. Each of the other five zones are occupied by one of the five viscera and five bowels. Thus there are 13 acuzones as shown on the figure above.

There are Eight Regions and 13 Acuzones:
I region: zone 1-Lung & zone 2-Large Intestine
II region: zone 3-Kidney & zone 4-Urinary Bladder
III region: zone 5-Upper Burner
IV region: zone 6-Liver & zone 7-Gallbladder
V region: zone 8-Middle Burner
VI region: zone 9-Heart & zone 10-Small Intestine
VII region: zone 11-Spleen & zone 12-Stomach
VIII region: zone13-Lower Burner

Note: Regions III, V and VIII only have one zone. This means that the upper, middle, and lower burners each occupy one region.

Treatment method

The upper and lower burner zones are chosen on the paralyzed side of the body. One should also consider using these same zones on the healthy side of the body if the patient's health condition is strong enough to take more needles. Prof. Peng used a 0.5 inch, 29 gauge needle. In the United States, I would suggest choosing smaller 32-38 gauge needles depending on the patient's tolerance to needles. The eyeball is stabilized by the pressing hand of the acupuncturist while the insertion hand inserts the needle horizontally into the appropriate zone, 2-5mm away from the edge of the orbit. (On the superior orbit, the insertion is above the edge. On the inferior orbit, the insertion is below the edge). Needles are retained for 10-20 minutes without manipulation. If the patient's condition allows, he or she should be encouraged to sit up. Then the practitioner should help the patient practice walking while the needles are still inserted around the eyes. To prevent bleeding after withdrawing the needles, one should apply pressure with a small cotton ball for at least three minutes to close the point.

The following summaries of three clinical trials conducted by Prof. Peng and his associates are examples of the effectiveness of this technique for the treatment of stroke.[10] In the first trial, 167 cases were treated with this method. Of those, 40 were basically cured, 66 registered a marked improvement, 56 got some improvement, and only five got no effect. Therefore, the total effectiveness rate was 97%. In the second study, 242 cases of stroke were treated by Prof. Peng and his associates.[11] Fifty-six of these cases were basically cured, 93 registered marked improvement, 87 got some improvement, and only five got no improvement. Therefore, the total effectiveness rate was 97.5%. In 1991 at the Liaoning College of Chinese Medicine, Dr. Zhu Feng-shan and his associates, under the direction of Professor Peng, completed a special clinical trial on the immediate response on raising the affected limb in stroke patients.[12] During 258 periocular treatments on 188 stroke patients, there were 221 treatments (85.66%) which indeed showed an immediate positive response on the raising of the paralyzed limb. In fact, only 37 patients or 14.36% did not show positive results. The main acuzones selected in this study were #5 upper burner and #13 lower burner bilaterally. The auxiliary acuzones selected consisted of #3 kidney, #6 liver, #7 gallbladder, and #9 heart, all on the affected side only. Needling techniques employed were done according to the methods used at Professor Peng's Ocular Acupuncture Research Center. The doctors observed the distance of increased movement of the affected upper limb by the distance it moved away from the chest and the ability to raise up the affected lower limb

from the treatment table before and right after treatment. If the result of the comparison was more than 10cm, it was counted as a positive response. Less than 10cm was counted as a negative response. These outcomes showed that periocular acupuncture can immediately accelerate the restoration of the motion of the paralyzed limbs in stroke patients.

According to Prof. Peng, the 12 regular channels all directly or indirectly connect to the area of the eye and, of course, also with all the viscera and bowels. The large intestine, stomach, gallbladder, small intestine, urinary bladder, and triple burner channels, along with internal branches of heart and liver channels all pass through the eye area. In addition, the internal-external relationship connects the lungs, spleen, kidneys, and pericardium indirectly to the areas around the eye. The reason for selecting the upper and lower burner zones is that these two areas are located at the inner and outer canthus, areas related to the yin and yang heel vessels, and the balance of these two vessels is beneficial for the motility of the body overall. This technique is safe, gentle, effective, and simple. It is especially good for patients at the onset of hemiplegia, yet can be effective in the rehabilitation phase as well. I have seen good results in my patients recovering from stroke after 1-2 years. I have also seen some improvement five years after stroke. The key still is, the sooner the treatment, the better the results. This method is easier for patients who are afraid of needles and who are too weak for longer treatment periods. Due to the short duration of this type of treatment and the location of needle insertion, it is unnecessary to remove any of the patient's clothing which is often a difficult process for stroke patients.

Shi Xue-min's Acupuncture Resuscitation Method for Stroke

Professor Shi Xue-min represented his study group from the First Hospital affiliated with Tianjin College of Chinese Medicine to present an article titled, "A Clinical Analysis & Experimental Study of 2336 Cases of Stroke Treated by the Acupuncture Resuscitation Method."[13] This study was conducted in 1987. At the Second World Conference of Acupuncture & Moxibustion in Paris held in November 1990, Dr. Li Guan[14] presented the following article summarized below, adding more updated data. After his presentation, I had a chance to speak with him personally. We discussed the details and methods he used as well as his integration of both Chinese and Western medicine. I was very impressed with the clinical studies and the integration he had done. I believe that this is the direction in which acupuncture science should be heading in the 21st century. In this section, I will introduce Prof. Shi's techniques and the outcomes of the above clinical trials. In Chapter 7, Dr. Peter Lau will discuss how these integrate with Western science.

In these trials, the main points consisted of *Ren Zhong* (GV 26), *Nei Guan* (Per 6), and *San Yin Jiao* (Sp 6). *Ren Zhong* was inserted obliquely to a depth of 0.5 inches below the nasal septum with supplementation technique and sparrow-pecking method. *Nei Guan* was inserted perpendicularly to a depth of 1-1.5 inches using lifting, thrusting, and rotating method and draining technique. For *San Yin Jiao*, oblique insertion was used with a depth of 0.8-1.0 inches with the tip of the needle resting right under the edge of tibia. Draining technique was used at *San Yin Jiao*. The auxiliary points consisted of *Ji Quan* (Ht 1), *Chi Ze* (Lu 5), *He Gu* (LI 4), and *Wei Zhong* (Bl 40). Draining technique was used at all these points along with the lifting and thrusting method. The effectiveness rate using this resuscitation method was 76.7% compared to 36.7% with traditional acupuncture methods. In addition, these outcomes have been substantiated and explained by electrophysiological studies and animal experiments. Using hemorrheology, it was shown that the viscosity of both whole blood and blood plasma decreased after treatment. Likewise, the volume of red cells after being centrifuged decreased after treatment. Further, electrophoresis of both red blood cells and platelets showed that they moved faster after treatment, and finally, agglutination of platelets decreased after treatment. In the comparison group treated with more a more regular selection of acupuncture points, there was little change in these parameters.

Prof. Shi and his research group continue to use and study this method. In 1992, an updated article was published in issue #1 of the *International Journal of Clinical Acupuncture*. The title of this article was, "Refreshment-Resuscitation Acupuncture for Cerebral Accidents (R-R Acupuncture)"The data in this study showed that another 871 stroke patients received the same method of treatment from 1987-1992. A total of 491 patients obtained a cure rate of 56.47%. The overall marked response rate was 79.64% (cure + marked response). The overall effectiveness rate was 98.47%. The average duration of patients' hospitalization was 45 days. In the past 15 years, this method has been used widely in China and there have been numerous clinical and laboratory studies reporting excellent results by treating stroke using this method.

Endnotes

[1] Yu Hui-chuan *et al.*, "Dr. Wang Le-ting's 13 Treatment Methods for Stroke," Beijing Shi Lao Zhong Yi Jing Yan Xuan Bian, *(A Selection of Old Chinese Doctors' Experiences)*, Beijing, 1980, p. 634-643

[2] Jiao Shun-fa, translated by Su Zhi-hong, *Head Acupuncture*, Shanxi Publishing House, Taiyuan, China, p. 105-122

Jiao Shun-fa, *Scalp Needling Therapy*, edited & translated by P. S. Yau, Medicine & Health Publishing Co. Hong Kong, 1984, p.36-38

[3] Chen Dao-yi *et al.*, "The Treatment of 444 Cases of Cerebral Paralysis & Aphasia Treated by Scalp Acupuncture," *Zhong Guo Zhen Jiu (Chinese Acupuncture & Moxibustion)*, #2, 1987, p. 9-10

[4] Wang Wen-yong, "Scalp Acupuncture in Treating Hemiplegia: Clinical Experiences with 24 Cases," *International Journal of Clinical Acupuncture*, Allerton Press, Inc., New York, U.S.A. 1996, Vol.7, No.4, p.463-465

[5] Wu Cheng-xun, et al., "Clinical Observations on the Treatment of 1228 Cases of Hemiplegia with Scalp Acupuncture," *Zhong Guo Zhen Jiu (Chinese Acupuncture & Moxibustion)*, #4, 1989, p. 3-5

[6] In the original article printed in Chinese, 12 treatments equaled one course for group II. I have assumed this was a typographical error because it does not make sense in comparison with groups I and III.

[7] Zhu Ming-qing, translated by Dale Chow King & Zheng Yuan-sheng, *Zhu's Scalp Acupuncture*, Eight Dragons Publishing, Hong Kong, Chinese Scalp Acupuncture Center of U.S.A., 1992

[8] Peng Jin-shan, *Eye Acupuncture Therapy*, Liaoning Science & Technology Publishing, Shenyang, China, 1990, p. 26-36

[9] Chan, Hoy Ping Yee, *Window of Health - Ocular Diagnosis and Periocular Acupuncture*, Northwest Institute of Acupuncture & Oriental Medicine, Seattle, WA, 1996, p. 39-44

[10] Peng Jin-shan *et al.*, "Clinical Observation on 167 Cases of Wind Stroke with Eye (Periocular) Acupuncture as Primary Method of Treatment," *Zhong Guo Zhen Jiu (Chinese Acupuncture & Moxibustion)*, #6, 1987, p. 23-24

[11] Peng Jin-shan, *op. cit.*, p. 92-94

[12] Zhu Feng-shan et al., "Observation on the Immediate Response from Using Periocular Acupuncture for Apoplectic Hemiplegia," *Zhong Guo Zhen Jiu (Chinese Acupuncture & Moxibustion)*, #3, 1991, p. 1921

[13] Shi Xue-min, "Observation of Hemorheology Changes & Effects on Stroke Patients at Acute Stage Treated by Resuscitation Method," *Compilation of the Abstracts of Acupuncture and Moxibustion* papers, First World Conference on Acupuncture—Moxibustion, Beijing, 1987, p. 36. Also *Zhong Guo Zhen Jiu (Chinese Acupuncture & Moxibustion)*, 1987, #1, p. 13

[14] Li Jun & Shi Xue-min, " Acupuncture in Apoplexy", *Second World Conference on Acupuncture & Moxibustion*, World Federation of Acupuncture Moxibustion Societies, Paris, 1990, p. 86

FOUR
Clinical Trials of the Treatment of Stroke Using Various Traditional Acupuncture Methods

In compiling this work, I have studied more than 50 articles published in *Zhong Guo Zhen Jiu* (*Chinese Acupuncture & Moxibustion*) from 1982 to 1994 as well as other Chinese acupuncture journals concerning the treatment of stroke. In this chapter, I discuss those articles involving different traditional acupuncture methods used to treat stroke which report similar effective results.

Treatment Based on Pattern Discrimination

In the two articles presented in this section, both predicate treatment based on Chinese medical pattern discrimination. Therefore, patients presenting different patterns received different groups of points. In the first study, 480 patients suffering from post-stroke hemiplegia were divided into five different patterns.[1]

1. Attack of the channels by wind with external evils still retained in the body

Patients presenting this pattern received acupuncture at *He Gu* (LI 4), *Wai Guan* (TB 5), *Tou Wei* (St 8), and *Feng Chi* (GB 20) using directional supplementation and drainage method. This is an acupuncture technique whereby the needle is angled either with or against the flow of the qi in the channel which produces supplementation or draining depending on that direction.[2] This technique only uses superficial puncture into the skin.

2. Vacuity of yin with repletion of yang, especially liver-gallbladder fire flaring upward

Patients presenting this pattern were treated with network vessel pricking (*i.e.*, bleeding) at *Bai Hui* (GV 20), *Tai Chong* (Liv 3), *Xia Xi* (GB 43), and *Tai Xi* (Ki 3).

3. Vacuity of liver-kidney yin as well as generalized yin and yang vacuity

Patients presenting this pattern were either needled deeply or received moxibustion at *Shen Shu* (Bl 23), *Tai Xi* (Ki 3), *Ming Men* (GV 4), and *San Yin Jiao* (Sp 6).

4. Spleen-kidney yang vacuity with phlegm and stasis in the channels

Patients presenting this pattern were either needled deeply or received moxibustion at *Zhong Wan* (CV 12), *Feng Long* (St 40), *Zu San Li* (St 36), and *San Yin Jiao* (Sp 6).

5. Qi & blood vacuity with malnourishment of the sinews and vessels

Patients presenting this pattern were needled at *Zu San Li* (St 36), *San Yin Jiao* (Sp 6), *Yang Ling Quan* (GB 34), and *Pi Shu* (Bl 20) or deep puncture was applied directly into the tendons of the rigid extremities without retaining the needles.

Of the 480 cases described in this article, 211 cases (43.95%) were cured, 136 cases got a marked effect, and 113 cases improved. Therefore, the total effectiveness rate was reported as 95.85%.

The second study in this section describes 108 cases of post-stroke hemiplegia.[3] Seventy-nine of these cases were diagnosed with infarction and 29 cases with hemorrhage in the brain. In this study, patients were divided into three patterns.

1. Phlegm stagnation with hemiplegia, profuse, sticky saliva and phlegm, a stiff tongue and unclear speech, dizziness, headache, white, slimy tongue fur, and a slippery pulse

Patients presenting this pattern were needled at *Pi Shu* (Bl 20), *Feng Long* (St 40), and *Gong Sun* (Sp 4).

2. Liver-kidney yin vacuity with rigid-type hemiplegia, a red facial complexion, tinnitus, constipation, a red tongue with yellow fur, and a bowstring, fast pulse

Patients presenting this pattern were nee-

dled at *Shen Shu* (Bl 23), *Fu Liu* (Ki 7), and *Tai Xi* (Ki 3).

3. Qi vacuity & blood stasis with flaccid-type hemiplegia, sallow yellow skin, edema of the extremities, a purple tongue body and/or static spots, and a fine pulse

Patients presenting this pattern were needled at *Qu Chi* (LI 11), *He Gu* (LI 4), and *Zu San Li* (St 36).

Additionally, some auxiliary points may have been added for local symptoms or scalp-needles were occasionally used with electrical stimulation.

In general, rather remarkable improvements were reported using the above protocol. Myodynamia increased more than two degrees after treatment in 23 cases, while myodynamia increased 1-2 degrees in 67 cases, with only 18 cases reporting no change. Total effectiveness was reported as 88.3%.

Treatment Based on Paralytic Site

In 1984, I supervised the internship of students of the Northwest Institute of Acupuncture & Oriental Medicine at the Chinese Medicine Research Institute of Chongqing City. It gave me a chance to learn more about the effect of acupuncture on stroke patients. This hospital had set up a research study team of 14 doctors who had training in both traditional Chinese medicine and modern Western medicine. The team was headed by Dr. Zheng Ban-tsan, with Dr. Wang Ji-gang as one of the main members of the team. This team published the following research in *Zhong Guo Zhen Jiu (Chinese Acupuncture &*

Moxibustion).[4]
For sequelae affecting the upper extremity, *Jian Yu* (LI 15), *Qu Chi* (LI 11), *He Gu* (LI 4), and *Wai Guan* (TB 5) were selected.

For sequelae affecting the lower extremity, *Huan Tiao* (GB 30), *Yang Ling Quan* (GB 34), *Zu San Li* (St 36), and *Xuang Zhong* (GB 39) were selected.

For deviation of eye and mouth, *Feng Chi* (GB 20), *Jia Che* (St 6), *Di Cang* (St 4), and *Wai Guan* (TB 5) were selected.

For aphasia, *Feng Chi* (GB 20) and *Lian Quan* (CV 23) were selected.

For vertigo due to hypertension, *Tai Chong* (Liv 3) and *Yong Quan* (Ki 1) were selected.

For weakness of the lumbar region, *Shen Shu* (Bl 23) and *Zu San Li* (St 36) were selected.

For emergency treatment, points were selected based on whether the patient presented tense or flaccid type symptoms.

For tense symptoms, *Shi Xuan* (M-HN-1) were pricked to bleed.[5] Then *Ren Zhong* (GV 26), *He Gu* (LI 4), and *Tai Chong* (Liv 3) were needled with draining technique.

For flaccid symptoms, *Shen Que* (CV 8) was indirectly moxaed over with salt and ginger. Moxibustion was also used on *Bai Hui* (GV 20), *Guan Yuan* (CV 4), *Zu San Li* (St 36), and *Yong Quan* (Ki 1).

Basic cure meant that the motor function of the paralyzed extremity basically recovered. Myodynamia was improved 4-5 degrees, and the patient was able to take care of him- or herself. Any facial paralysis or speech problems also disappeared. Marked

effect meant that the motor function of the paralyzed extremity showed a marked recovery. Improvement in myodynamia increased 3-4 degrees. Facial paralysis was markedly improved, and the patient was basically able to take care of him- or herself. Improvement meant that the motor function of the extremity had improved somewhat. Myodynamia had increased one degree, but the patient still could not walk without assistance. No effect meant that, after treatment, the patient's symptoms had remained unchanged. Based on these criteria, 89 cases (35.5%) were basically cured, 73 cases (29.1%) got a marked effect, 81 cases (32.2%) improved somewhat, and only eight cases (3.2%) got no effect. Therefore, the total effectiveness rate was reported as 96.8%.

A number of things were also concluded from this study based on the experiences of the research team.[6] First, emergency treatment should be started as soon as possible. Sometimes acupuncture was started as soon as patients arrived in the emergency room. Of course, to save the patient's life, they combined Western medical treatment with acupuncture. Secondly, for the prevention of sequelae, time is important. Acupuncture treatment should start as soon as possible to stop the pathological mechanisms responsible for the causation of sequelae. For this purpose, the research team developed a three-step protocol:

1. Free the flow of the channels and regulate the qi and blood.
2. Arouse the spleen, and boost the qi.
3. Strengthen the patient's righteous qi and support their original or source qi.

Clinical results in the above treatment group varied with their start dates. For patients receiving acupuncture within three months of their strokes, the rate of cure was 41.5%. For patients who began acupuncture four months after their strokes, the cure rate was only 1.3%. This clearly means that the sooner treatment begins, the better the results.

It is very important too that the extremities be exercised during treatment. In some cases, even though the myodynamia had already shown recovery, the patient still experienced weakness while standing or walking. Fortifying the spleen and supplementing the qi is effective for improving this. In this case, light stimulation was administered at *Zhong Wan* (CV 12), *Guan Yuan* (CV 4), and *Zu San Li* (St 36). Although the results demonstrated the effectiveness of acupuncture for the sequela of both ischemic and hemorrhagic infarction, the effectiveness rate was much higher for the ischemic infarction group. While the muscle tone is recovering, the muscles may show some rigidity on the flexor side. In that case, one should choose some points on yin channels and also directly puncture the tendons to relieve the rigidity. Further, a wide selection of points, light stimulation, and long retention of needles are beneficial in some cases. In general, points should mainly be chosen on the yang ming channels. In some cases, the combination of body needles and scalp acupuncture should be given. In that case, body needling should be carried out once daily, and scalp acupuncture should be done twice weekly. Such combination treatment is especially good for the upper extremities. After withdrawing the needles, moxibustion using a moxa stick can be added to increase the regulation and rectification of the qi and blood. In a few cases, long-term acupuncture may cause some pain and numbness in the extremities. This is due to blood vacuity and may be prevented by prescribing Chinese herbs to both nourish and quicken the blood.

Traditional Acupuncture Treatment With Emphasis on Manual Manipulation Methods

In order to obtain better results for stroke survivors, many acupuncturists have tried very hard to improve their hand techniques, meaning the way the needles are manipulated after insertion. In this section, I discuss two different studies where the choice and implementation of various hand techniques is considered extremely important for the outcomes. The author of the first study believes that, although the same points might be selected for the treatment of paralysis due to stroke, if they present different patterns, these points should be manipulated with different hand techniques. In this study, the author treated 148 cases of post-stroke hemiplegia.[7] Of these, 91 were male and 57 were female. These patients' ages ranged from 32-78 years of age, with an average age of 57.3. The points selected consisted of the five back transport points plus *Feng Fu* (GV 16), *Bai Hui* (GV 20), *He Gu* (LI 4), *Jian Yu* (LI 15), *Huang Tiao* (GB 30), and *Yang Ling Quan* (GB 34). However, two different hand techniques were employed.

1. Green dragon moving its tail

The needle was inserted to obtain the qi. Then the needle was withdrawn upward to the surface level of the point. The needle was next pushed flat under the skin. Then the handle of the needle was moved back and forth to the left and right at a 45 degree angle 9-27 times until the patient felt increased distention. Then the needle was slowly withdrawn, after which the point was quickly closed. This method was used for cases with a root vacuity. For symptoms of repletion, points were needled with the supplementation on the healthy side and drainage on the paralyzed side.

2. White tiger shaking its head

The needle was first inserted deeply to obtain the qi. Then, using two fingers to stabilize the handle of the needle and following the patient's breathing, the needle was twisted further in and shaken to the left. During inhalation, the needle was withdrawn and shaken to the right. This hand technique was selected for cases of repletion.

Usually, the patient was treated once a day, with 10 treatments equaling one course. Treatments continued for 2-3 courses. If the stroke had happened more than one month prior to treatment, the patient was seen every other day for 5-6 courses or a total of 50-60 treatments. After this time, 57 cases were cured, 56 cases got a marked effect, 27 cases got some effect, and six cases got no effect. Two cases became worse. Therefore, the total effectiveness rate was 94.6%.

In the second study, the author emphasized the use of different hand techniques in different stages of the treatment of stroke patients.[8] In his opinion, patients' post-stroke pathologies vary with the amount of time since their stroke. Thus different treatment methods are needed. Therefore, the author divided the patients in this study into three different treatment stages. Altogether, there were 919 males and 701 females 19-82 years of age in this study totaling 1,620 cases. However, the majority of patients were 50-60 years old. Treatment began as early as two days after the initial stroke to as late as three years after. There were 893 cases of left-sided paralysis and 727 cases of right-sided paralysis. One thousand three hundred forty-two cases were diagnosed with ischemic infarction, and 278 cases

were diagnosed with hemorrhagic infarction. These 1,620 patients were randomly divided into two groups. There were 972 cases in the treatment group, and 648 cases in the comparison group.

All members of the treatment group received acupuncture according to which of the three stages post-stroke they were in. Those in the early stage (*i.e.*, within six months of their stroke) were needled on their healthy side while their paralyzed side was mobilized. This idea comes from the *Zhen Jin Da Cheng (Great Compendium of Acupuncture & Moxibustion)*. According to this text the healthy side has a repletion of qi, and the paralyzed side has a vacuity of qi. Needling on the healthy side drains the repletion and frees the flow of the channels.

For those whose stroke occurred 6-18 months previous, needles were inserted bilaterally to keep the body in balance. According to the author, qi vacuity and blood stasis are the main disease mechanisms present in this stage. For patients 1.5-3 years post-stroke, running needle technique was used along with fire needle in the cases of vacuity, while bleeding was used in cases of repletion. All members of the comparison group were needled on the paralyzed side to regulate and warm the channels. All patients in both groups were treated once a day, with 10 treatments equaling a course . Following a three day rest, treatment was then resumed for another course. All patients in both groups were needled at the same points: *Qu Chi* (LI 11), *Nei Guan* (Per 6), *He Gu* (LI 4), *Bai Hui* (GV 20), *Zu San Li* (St 36), *Yang Ling Quan* (GB 34), and *San Yin Jiao* (Sp 6).

The results from this showed a remarkable difference in outcome between those in the early stage subgroup of the treatment group and those in the comparison group in the early stage of treatments. The cure rate of the early stage patients in the treatment group was 47.2%, while it was only 30.66% in the comparison group. In the middle stage subgroup, the cure rate was 37.74%, compared to only 24.88% in the comparison group. This was also a remarkable difference. There were no cured cases in the late stage subgroup or in the comparison group. The total effectiveness rate was 72.33% in the treatment group but only 48.65% in the comparison group. This was also a significant statistical difference. Based on these outcomes, it was concluded that altering treatment based on the above three stages of disease is more effective than simply giving the same acupuncture treatment regardless of how long ago the stroke had occurred.

Endnotes

[1] Wang Xin-ming, "Clinical Observations on the Acupuncture Treatment of 480 Cases of Hemiplegia," *Zhong Guo Zhen Jiu (Chinese Acupuncture & Moxibustion)*, #6, 1986, p. 5-6

[2] Needling with the tip pointing in the direction of the channel flow produces supplementation, whereas needling with the tip pointing counter to the direction of the flow produces drainage. Wiseman, Nigel & Feng Ye, *Introduction to English Terminology of Chinese Medicine*, Paradigm Publications, Brookline, MA, 2002, p. 245

[3] Fang You-an, *et al.*, "Relationship Between the Effect of Acupuncture on Apopletic Hemiplegia and Computed Tomography—An Analysis of 108 Cases," *Shang Hai Zhen Jiu Za Zhi (Shanghai Journal of Acupuncture & Moxibustion)*, #4, 1989, p. 1

[4] Wang Ji-gang, *et al.*, "Clinical Observations on the Acupuncture Treatment of 251 Cases of the Sequelae of Stroke," *Zhong Guo Zhen Jiu (Chinese Acupuncture & Moxibustion)*, #6, 1987, p. 18-19

[5] *Shi Xuan* (M-HN-1): A set of 10 points, one on the middle of the tip of each finger, about 0.1 unit from the fingernail.

[6] These remarks were mostly given by Shou-chun Ma, L.Ac., M.TCM, an acupuncturist who formally worked with the stroke research study team in Chongqing Institute of TCM, Sichuan Province, China. He now runs a private acupuncture clinic and practices in Seattle, WA.

[7] Gu Yu-xin, "Using Traditional Hand Techniques for Hemiplegia—148 Cases," *Zhong Guo Zhen Jiu (Chinese Acupuncture & Moxibustion)*, #5, 1990, p. 4

[8] Wang Hang-zhi, *et al.*, "Clinical Observation of Acupuncture Treating 1,620 Cases of Paraplegia," *Zhong Guo Zhen Jiu (Chinese Acupuncture & Moxibustion)*, #6, 1991, p. 1-2

FIVE
Clinical Trials Exemplifying the Use of Special Techniques

This chapter contains a survey of 23 clinical trials using treatment methods not typically included in textbooks. Among more than 60 articles reviewed, we selected those studies with 1) large cohorts, 2) conducted by doctors, 3) who worked in larger or more famous facilities, and 4) those presenting the most unique treatment methods. Hopefully, the introduction of these special techniques will provide practitioners with more treatment options for gaining the utmost effects in their practice. However, some of the techniques included in this chapter are not easy to do and may have risky side effects if not done properly. Therefore, practitioners wishing to employ these riskier techniques should learn them from someone who has experience in those techniques.

One Point Treatment[1]

In this clinical trial, there were 138 males and 59 females. Five cases were under 30 years old, nine cases were 30-40 years old, 37 cases were 41-50 years old, 82 cases were 51-60 years old, 53 cases were 61-70 years old, and 11 cases were over 71 years old. One hundred twenty-eight of these cases

received treatment within one year of the onset of stroke, 43 received treatment within 1-5 years, while 26 were treated 5-11 years after the onset of their stroke. *Ren Ying* (St 9) was needled bilaterally on all these patients. The depth of needle insertion varied with the diameter of the patient's neck. Insertion was 2-2.5 centimeters deep on those necks which were 29-34 centimeters in diameter and was 2.5-4 centimeters deep for those whose necks were 35-42 centimeters in diameter.[2] With the patient in supine position, the acupuncturist used his or her index finger to locate the pulse of the carotid artery, pushing the superior jugular vein to the side. After disinfecting the skin at this point, he or she first quickly inserted a 28 gauge filiform needle into the skin and then slowly went deeper at the point until the patient felt numbness, distention, and heaviness. The needle was slightly rotated for 1-2 minutes. The tip of the needle was angled toward the affected side of the body until the arrival of qi to that area. Then the needle was withdrawn. There was no passive retention of the needles. Ten treatments equaled one course of treatment. In addition, all patients were administered vessel-dilating medications as part of their basic care. Using this technique, 54 cases (27.4%) were cured,

61 cases (30.9%) experienced a marked effect, 75 cases (38.1%) improved, and only seven cases (3.6%) got no effect. Therefore, the total effectiveness rate was 96.4%.

Ren Ying is located on the yang ming channel which has lots of qi and lots of blood. Eight channels meet at this point: the lung, spleen, stomach, heart, kidney, triple burner, gallbladder, and small intestine channels. Needling *Ren Ying* balances yin and yang, moves the qi and dispels stasis, thus promoting the body's recovery. Before using *Ren Ying*, the acupuncturist *must* be familiar with its location and anatomy as well as follow clean needle technique. The patient should be put in a suitable position and the practitioner should avoid piercing the artery and vein. The needle insertion and manipulation should be very careful. In case of bleeding, apply pressure to stop the bleeding and avoid hematoma.[3] Dr. Wu's team used this method for more that 10,000 treatments without side effects.

Selecting Points Only on the Yang Ming[4]

The yang ming channels contain lots of qi and lots of blood. Therefore, using acupoints on these channels can regulate and rectify both the qi and blood, and, as we have seen above, the qi and blood are both closely related to the disease mechanisms of stroke. The following clinical trial examines the effects of using only acupoints on the yang ming channels to treat stroke patients. All 60 patients in this study were diagnosed by cranial CT scan as well as by Chinese medical practitioners. The degree of disability was categorized from class 0-VII.[5] Forty of the patients were male and 20 were female. Their average age was 63. The

shortest time from the onset of stroke was 29 days and the longest was 160 days. These 60 patients were randomly divided into two groups: a treatment group and a comparison group, with 30 patients each. All patients were administered acupuncture beginning the day after their admission to the hospital. Further, blood rheology[6] and cranial blood flow (TCD)[7] were examined on all subjects before administering acupuncture.

In the treatment group, patients were treated with acupoints selected solely on the yang ming. The points consisted of *He Gu* (LI 4), *Shou San Li* (LI 10), *Qu Chi* (LI 11), *Jian Yu* (LI 15), *Bi Guan* (St 31), *Fu Tu* (St 32), *Zu San Li* (St 36), and *Jie Xi* (St 41). Members of the comparison group were needled at *Wai Guan* (TB 5), *Jian Liao* (TB 14), *Chi Ze* (Lu 5), *Hou Xi* (SI 3), *Huan Tiao* (GB 30), *Feng Shi* (GB 31), *Yang Ling Quan* (GB 34), and *Kun Lun* (Bl 60).

Additions and subtractions were the same for both groups. For speech difficulties, *Ya Men* (GV 15) and *Shang Lian Quan* (M-HN-21)[11] were added. For deviation of the mouth, *Xia Guan* (St 7) and *Di Cang* (St 4) were added. All patients in both groups received acupuncture once per day with the needles retained for 30 minutes each time. The needles were manipulated using supplementing hand technique. Ten days equaled one course of treatment, and there was no break between each successive course. All patients were re-evaluated after three treatment series.

Basic cure and the total effectiveness rates were 36.67% and 96.67% respectively in the treatment group, and 6.67% and 80.00% respectively in the comparison group. Thus there was statistically significant difference in efficacy between the two groups after the treatment (P<0.005). With reference to the blood rheology, there was no significant differences between treatment and comparison groups before treatment (P>0.5), but there were noticeable differences between the two groups after the treatment (P<0.05). With the cranial blood flow, there were noticeable differences between the before and after treatment in the treatment group (P<0.01), while no significant differences appeared in the control group (0.1<P<0.25). In their discussion, the authors of this study begin by saying that qi and blood are closely related to stroke. In the Ming dynasty, Wang Lun stated in Ming Yi Za Zha *(Ming Medical Miscellany)*, that qi vacuity, qi stagnation, blood vacuity, and blood stasis are all factors causing stroke. Further, in the chapter titled "On Wind," he said:

> Human blood circulates in the blood vessels and fills up the skin and hair externally. It infiltrates the muscles and nourishes the sinews and bones. Therefore, if there is harmony [of the blood in the body], there is no difficulty in daily activities. If qi is stagnant, blood will become static; if the qi counterflows, blood will counterflow as well. When combined with heat, stagnation and turbidity will result. When combined with cold, clotting will result.

In the "Paralysis Chapter" of the Qing dynasty book, *Yi Lin Gai Cuo (Correcting the Errors in the Forest of Medicine)*, it is mentioned that stroke is caused by damage of the original qi. When qi and blood are damaged, the channels and networks become vacuous and qi will then circulate on one side only, thus causing paralysis. Therefore, treatment should focus on regulating the qi and blood. Hence, in ancient times, it was said:

> To treat wind, first treat the blood. When the blood moves, wind is automatically extinguished.

And,

> Qi is the commander of blood. When the qi moves, the blood moves.

There is also a close relationship between the yang ming channels and the function of the limb. Because the yang ming has lots of blood and the blood nourishes the sinews, the yang ming also controls the sinews. Thus it is said, "When the yang ming is vacuous, the sinews are slack." Further, when the sinews are slack, they cannot control the bones nor disinhibit the joints. Thus, the normal functions of the muscles and limbs depend on the nourishment of the qi and blood via these channels. In addition, acupoints on the yang ming channels also fortify and boost the spleen and stomach. Since the spleen and stomach are the latter heaven root of qi and blood transformation and engenderment, needling points on these channels supplements the qi and nourishes the blood of the entire body. Because the qi moves the blood and the blood nourishes the vessels, insuring that the qi and blood are exuberant helps promote the free flow through the channels and vessels. Therefore, this technique not only treats the root but also the branches or tips of this condition. The root causes are liver-kidney yin vacuity, profuse phlegm and accumulation of dampness, yang qi vacuity, and former heaven natural endowment insufficiency. The tip or branch causes include traumatic injury, such as accidental fall and contusion, exhaustion, emotional excitement, excessive exertion, and contraction of external evils. The tip or branch causes can also be triggered by the root causes.

And finally, according to modern research,

needling acupoints on the yang ming channels has a homeostatic or regulatory function on the blood flow in the cranial arteries. Needling these points can both speed up the arterial blood flow when the flow is too slow and slow down the arterial blood flow when flow is too rapid. Recent studies have also shown that needling *Zu San Li* (St 36) can constrict blood vessels that are too dilated or dilates blood vessels which are too constricted. Such homeostatic regulation is probably due to the regulation of the alpha-receptors in the large blood vessels and the beta-receptors in the small blood vessels in the neural-body fluid system. As a result, both the viscosity and the permeability of blood are regulated which then limits the formation and spread of thrombosis. Thus acupuncture on the yang ming points improves the supply of blood and oxygen to the affected areas and helps restore their neural functions.

Running Needles Technique on the Yin Channels[8]

Using running needles on points located on the yin channels increases the intensity of stimulation and, at the same time, regulates imbalances of viscera in order to treat root disease mechanisms. In the two-wing comparison study described below, there were 162 patients in the treatment group. Of these, 108 were male and 54 were female. The youngest was 50 years old, while the oldest was 78. Of the total patients, 128 subjects had suffered a stroke within three months prior to commencement of treatment. In the comparison group of 54 patients, 38 were male and 16 were female. Their ages ranged from 42-76 years. Forty-nine of the patients in the comparison group were treated within three months of suffering stroke. All members of the treatment group received running needle acupuncture

at the following pairs of points:

Ji Quan (Ht 1)[9] ⟶ *Jian Yu* (LI 15)
Chi Ze (Lu 5) ⟶ *Shao Hai* (Ht 3)
Nei Guan (Per 6) ⟶ *Wai Guan* (TB 5)
He Gu (LI 4) ⟶ *Lao Gong* (Per 8)
Ci Liao (Bl 32) ⟶deep insertion to the front part of perineum[10]
Yin Ling Quan (Sp 9)⟶*Yang Ling Quan* (GB 34)
San Yin Jiao (Sp 6) ⟶ *Xuan Zhong* (GB 39)
Tai Chong (Liv 3) ⟶*Yong Quan* (Ki 1)

If there was deviation of the mouth and eye, *Di Cang* (St 4) through to *Jia Che* (St 6) was added. If there was loss of speech, *Shang Lian Quan* (M-HN-21) through to the root of the tongue was added.[11] For unconsciousness, *Ren Zhong* (GV 26) and *Yi Feng* (TB 17) were added. After the qi was obtained, electrical stimulation was applied to the paired needles using the dense-disperse wave form frequency.[12] The stimulation used was the maximum that the patient could tolerate. Electro-acupuncture was performed for 30 minutes once per day. Ten days of treatments equaled one course, with 3-5 days rest between each successive course. During these acupuncture treatments, the subjects were closely monitored with functional training. All members of the comparison group were needled at *Qu Chi* (LI 11), *Jian Yu* (LI 15), *Wai Guan* (TB 5), *He Gu* (LI 4), *Huan Tiao* (GB 30), *Zu San Li* (St 36), *Xuan Zhong* (GB 39), and *Tai Chong* (Liv 3). Auxiliary points were the same as the treatment group as was electrical stimulation and the length of treatments.[12] Likewise, physical exercises during treatment was the same.

The results were classified into four categories.[13] The cure and total effectiveness rates[14] were 64% and 97% respectively in the treatment group, but only 41% and 85%

respectively in the comparison group (P<0.01). These differences were statistically significant. This study also showed that the total effectiveness rate was higher for those subjects who received acupuncture treatments within three months following their stroke compared to those who received treatment after three months had passed (P<0.01).

Because the authors of this study believe there is a close relationship between the pathogenesis of stroke and imbalance of the viscera, especially the heart, spleen, liver, and kidneys, they mainly needled acupoints on the yin channels to regulate the functions of the five viscera. This was considered a root treatment. According to these authors, running needles promote the communication between the external and internal as well as the qi in the two related channels. Running needle technique not only increases the intensity of stimulation and the extent of the stimulated area but also stimulates the qi of the whole body, freeing the flow of the constructive and defensive, the qi and blood throughout the body. Hence, the neural function was restored and the healing process was speeded up. This study also showed that, the earlier acupuncture treatments were started following the onset of stroke, the higher the effectiveness of the treatments. In addition, from the CT scanning of certain subjects, it was found that the efficacy of treatment was also closely related to the location of pressure and blockage.

Prescription based on the flow of qi in the 12 channels[15]

A large benefit of this technique is that it uses a choice of either a one-needle or three-needle treatment. Additionally, the method is especially good for the treatment of ischemic cases and early stroke treatment in order to increase blood flow to the brain. In this study, Ma Dan-yang's leverage-interception acupoint selection method was used.[16] This method was first introduced in the Song dynasty in Ma Dan-yang's Tian Xing Shi Er Xue Dan Chuo Fa (*The Song of the Twelve Heavenly Star Points for the Treatment of Disease*). Leverage in the name of this technique refers to selecting two acupoints on each side of the upper limb or one point on the upper limb and another point on the lower limb on one side of the body. This is likened to the action of a lever. "Interception" refers to selecting only one acupoint on a limb, using it to stop the progress of the symptoms. One of the benefits of this technique is that it uses either only one needle or, at most, three needles per treatment. Thus pain due to needling is minimal. Additionally, the method is especially good for the treatment of ischemic cases and early stroke treatment in order to increase blood flow to the brain. There were 176 stroke patients enrolled in this study. The patients were divided into two groups. The first group, 98 males and 34 females, were treated with the leverage-interception method. The second group, 25 males and 19 females, were treated with traditional acupuncture as a comparison group. In both groups, the youngest patient was 50 and the oldest was 65 years of age. These patients had suffered from stroke for at least seven days and up to 30 days prior to treatment. All the patients in both groups also received 20 milliliters of *Mai Luo Ling* (Vessel & Network Vessel Magically Effective [Medication]) in 250 milliliters of normal saline solution as an intravenous drip daily for 10 days in combination with the acupuncture. Speech, mobility, and neurological functions were tested before and after treatment. This was accompanied by examination in improvement of symptoms from a Chinese medical point of view. Other tests before and after treatment included hemodynamics and CT scan of blood flow in the brain.

According to the qi flow in 12 channels and the internal and external relationship of the channels, four groups of acupoint combinations were used in the treatment group. The first combination consisted of *Lei Que* (Lu 7) on the healthy side and *Qu Chi* (LI 11) on the affected side on the upper part of the body and *Zu San Li* (St 36) on the affected side on the lower part of the body. The second combination consisted of *He Gu* (LI 4) on affected side on the upper part of the body and *Nei Ting* (St 44) on affected side and *Kun Lun* (Bl 60) on the unaffected side of the lower part of the body. The third combination consisted of *Tong Li* (Ht 5) on affected side on the upper part of the body plus *Wei Zhong* (Bl 40) on affected side and *Cheng Shan* (Bl 57) on healthy side on the lower part of the body. Combination four consisted of *Yang Ling Quan* (GB 34), *Huan Tiao* (GB 30), and *Tai Chong* (Liv 3), all on the affected side. Only one of these points was used each time. Each of these combinations was used for five days, and acupuncture was administered once per day without supplementing or draining hand technique. The needles were retained in the body for 30 minutes per treatment and manipulated once after 15 minutes of retention. Twenty days of treatment equaled one course.

In the comparison group, *Feng Chi* (GB 20), *Jian Yu* (LI 15), *Qu Chi* (LI 11), *He Gu* (LI 4), *Wai Guan* (TB 5), *Huan Tiao* (GB 30), *Zu San Li* (St 36), *Xuan Zhong* (GB 39) and *Tai Chong* (Liv 3) were needled on the affected side. For speech difficulties, *Tong Li* (Ht 5) and *Lian Quan* (CV 23) were added. For contraction of the extremities, *Ba Feng* (M-LE-8) and *Hou Xi* (SI 3)

were added. Acupuncture was administered once per day without supplementation or drainage hand technique. The needles were retained in the body for 30 minutes each time and manipulated once after 15 minutes of retention. One course of treatment consisted of 20 days. In the treatment group, the total effectiveness rate was 92.5%, while the cure rate was 52.3%. In the comparison group, the total effectiveness and cure rates were 86.4% and 50.0% respectively. Further, there were remarkable improvements in speech and joint mobility using the leverage-interception method. However, in the comparison group, improvement rates in speech and joint mobility were not as marked (P > 0.05). Both groups showed significant effects in terms of hemodynamics. Increased cerebral blood flow in those treated with the leverage-interception method was better than in the comparison group after 15 minutes of treatment. However, there was no significant difference between the two groups after 20 days of treatment. According to the authors of this study, the causes of stroke are wind, phlegm, and/or blood stasis due to qi vacuity, and the symptoms of paralysis, speech impediment, and numbness are caused by unsmooth or uneasy flow of qi, disharmony of the channels and network vessels, and malnourishment of the channels and sinews. Because the leverage-interception method connects 12 acupoints, it promotes the circulation and regulates the qi and blood in the 12 channels. For example, qi and blood flow starts in the lung channel and ends in the liver channel. Then the qi and blood flow from the liver to the lung channel and the cycle repeats itself continuously. Using Ma Dan-yang's leverage-interception method, the flow of qi and blood is regulated from *Lie Que* to *Tai Chong*. In addition, among the 12 Heavenly Star points, nine points belong to the hand or foot yang channels. On the hand yang ming, there is *He Gu* (LI 4) and *Qu Chi* (LI 11). On the foot *yang ming*, there is *Zu San Li* (St 36) and *Nei Ting* (St 44). On the foot *tai yang*, we have *Wei Zhong* (Bl 40), *Cheng Shan* (Bl 57), and *Kun Lun* (Bl 60), and on the foot *shao yang*, we have *Huan Tiao* (GB 30) and *Yang Ling Chuan* (GB 34). Stroke patients commonly have motion or mobility problems. Since yang corresponds to active-ness and movement, using points from the yang channels to treat stroke patients with mobility problems makes sense according to the logic of Chinese medicine.

Paravertebral Point Needling[17]

In the following clinical trial, needling the paravertebral or *jia ji* points was combined with scalp acupuncture. Needling the par-avertebral points aids the circulation of the qi and blood locally as well as frees the flow of the channels. Scalp acupuncture improves the blood flow and oxygen supply in the cerebral cortex. All 100 patients were diagnosed by CT scan as having suffered a stroke. Of these, 64 were males and 36 were females. The youngest was 35, while the oldest was 83 years of age. However, most of the patients were 50-70 years of age. The shortest duration of from the onset of illness was three days and the longest was one year. The hemiplegia symptoms affected 68 subjects on the left side and 32 on the right. In terms of type of stroke, 72 patients had suffered cranial infarction, while 28 had suffered cranial hemorrhage. These patients were randomly divided into a treatment and comparison group of 50 patients each.

All members of the treatment group began treatment by laying on the unaffected side of the body while acupuncture of paraverte-bral points was carried out along the cervi-cal, thoracic, and lumbar regions. Insertion of the needles was 1-1.5 inches deep. After the qi was obtained, even supplementing-even draining hand technique was used. Scalp acupuncture was carried out on the motor area as well as on the motor and sen-sory area of the foot. The needles were inserted through the scalp to the subcuta-neous layer to a depth of 0.5-1 inch. Frequent twisting manipulation was per-formed at these points. During this treat-ment, the patients were encouraged to move the afflicted limbs.

All members of the comparison group began their treatment by lying in the prone posi-tion. Acupuncture was administered at *Da Zui* (GV 14) in addition to *Jian Wai Shu* (SI 14), *Qu Chi* (LI 11), *He Gu* (LI 4), *Wai Guan* (TB 5), *Yao Yang Guan* (GV 3), *Bai Huan Shu* (Bl 30), *Huan Tiao* (GB 30), *Yang Ling Quan* (GB 34), *Zu San Li* (St 36), *Jie Xi* (St 41), and *Kun Lun* (Bl 60) on the affected side of the body. After the qi was obtained, no further supplementing or drain-ing technique was used. Scalp acupuncture was the same as the treatment group. Acupuncture was administered once per day to both treatment and comparison groups, with 10 treatments equaling one course. Two days of rest were allowed between each successive course, and effectiveness was evaluated after six courses of treatment. Patients in both the treatment and compari-son groups were evaluated according to their muscular strength, extensibility, and mobility. The outcomes were classified as cured, marked effect, some effect, and no effect.[18] The total effectiveness rates[19] in the treatment and comparison groups were 94% and 84% respectively (P < 0.01). According to the authors of this study, Hua Tuo's par-avertebral points are extraordinary points. They lie between the governing vessel and the foot *tai yang* bladder channel.

Anatomically, each paravertebral point is associated with the dorsal rami of one of the spinal nerve plus its arteries and veins. Therefore, based on the Chinese medical theory that, "Associated diseases can be treated wherever the channel and network vessels pass through," needling the paravertebral points has multiple effects. These include freeing the flow of the channels, smoothing the circulation of qi and blood, as well as enhancing the local blood circulation and improving the nourishment to the surrounding tissues. Additionally, sympathetic nerves release several chemicals including bradykinin, 5-hydroxytryptamine, and acetylcholine. These improve the cranial supply of blood and oxygen. As a result, the collateral circulation in the cerebral arterial circle of the afflicted side can be enhanced and the nervous pathways of functional mobility can be restored. Scalp acupuncture, on the other hand, can reflexively increase the volume of blood flow as well as improve the oxygen supply in the cerebral cortex. As a result, the functions of the cortex can be restored. Thus needling the paravertebral points together with scalp acupuncture can enhance the collateral circulation in the cranial blood vessels with the effect that cranial thrombi or emboli are softened and cranial blood circulation is improved. As a result, blood supply to the brain is also improved. Additionally, it enhances the activity of the fibrinolysin system in the plasma. As a result of this, clots in the area of cerebral hemorrhage or cerebral thrombosis are dissolved faster along with decreased viscosity and agglutination in the blood. All these factors help to restore the bodily functions in hemiplegia.

Tongue Acupuncture

Currently, research is being conducted in China to understand the importance of using tongue acupuncture in the treatment of stroke and its complications or sequelae. In the article, "Indicators of Changes in Stroke Patients' Tongue Appearance for Differential Classification," the authors emphasize the importance of the tongue in traditional Chinese medical theory as a reflection of the human qi and the function of the viscera and bowels.[20] By looking at the tongue the practitioner can tell not only about the viscera and bowels but also how the patient is responding to treatment or if there are other avenues of treatment that might be beneficial. The authors offer nine classifications of tongues seen in stroke patients.

1. Stiff tongue
In this case, the speech is sluggish, primarily due to liver wind with phlegm attacking vessels around *Lian Quan* (CV 23). Ascendant liver yang hyperactivity obstructs and congests within the sinews and vessels, thus causing stiffness. Further breakdown of this classification indicates a light stroke if the patient slobbers or drools and cannot talk well. Also, light symptoms may indicate a TIA, while very strong symptoms indicate the acute stage of stroke. Stiff tongue is commonly seen in long-term patients and is difficult to treat successfully.

2. Crooked tongue
The tongue pulls towards the healthy side of the body when the patient sticks it out causing unclear speech and drooling. Crooked tongue is caused by wind phlegm stagnating in network vessels. If this type of tongue is still evident six months after stroke, it indicates a high chance of the stroke recurring. The possibility of another stroke is less if the whole body recovers and the crooked tongue improves.

3. Quivering tongue

Tremors are caused by qi and blood dual vacuity leading to yang vacuity, resulting in the tongue not being warmed and steamed. Resulting damage occurs leaving it unable to calm down. This condition is more common in elderly stroke patients. Quivering tongue indicates a difficult case and that it will take long-term treatment to achieve improvement.

4. Atrophied tongue

In this case, the tongue muscle has wasted away and has no strength due to a qi and yin dual vacuity in the sinews and vessels. The atrophy is worse on the same side as the stroke. The patient also experiences cold in the limbs and generalized fatigue.

5. & 6. Protruding/rigid tongue [21]

The tongue sticks out of the mouth and will not retract, thus indicating a serious stroke. This is caused either by qi vacuity or, more acutely, replete heat in the body causing phlegm and fire stirring in the heart. This tongue sign is not commonly seen but, in long-term stroke patients, it signals serious problems with the essence qi and offers little hope for recovery. It may even indicate impending death. A rigid or protruding tongue may also be seen in post-stroke patients with vascular dementia.

7. Darting tongue

The tongue moves rapidly and erratically in and out between the lips. Patients with this rare condition should be considered at high risk because it often signals an impending stroke. He/she should be given more tests and watched closely in case of the occurrence of stroke.

8. Numb tongue

The tongue, which is usually numb on the side of the body affected by the stroke, moves choppily. This is a common effect of stroke caused by yin-blood vacuity combined with wind phlegm. The patient loses their sensation of taste and, in severe cases, can easily bite their tongue when eating.

9. Contracted tongue

The tongue cannot stick out and speech is poor. This tongue sign may be due to vacuity, repletion, cold, or heat since many conditions contribute to it. This sign indicates a difficult-to-treat case of stroke. If the tongue both contracts and curls like a bowl, it indicates that the stroke patient is in a critical stage.

Locations & indications of basic and newly proposed lingual points important for the treatment of stroke[22]

Heart: This point is located at the tip of the tongue and treats the heart.

Kidneys: This point is located four *fen* lateral to the bladder and treats the bladder and kidneys.

Frontal: With the tongue tip pressed against the upper incisors, this point is located three *fen* behind the tip of the tongue on the inferior surface. It treats headache and vertigo.

Ju Quan: This point is located two *fen* in front of Stomach. This point is indicated for wasting thirst and tongue stiffness.

Upper limb: At margin of the tongue, between Lung and Gallbladder. It treats the upper limbs.

Lower limb: This point is located near the tongue margin, one *cun* lateral to Yin. It treats the lower limbs.

Jin Jin (**left**) *Yu Ye* (**right**): These two separately named points are located on the veins lateral to the frenulum. According to Bensky and O' Connor, they are M-HN-20.

They treat stomatitis, glossitis, pharyngitis, and vomiting.

She Zhu: This point is located on the inferior surface of the tongue. It treats double tongue and swollen tongue.

Zhong Ju: This point is located on the boundary between bottom of the tongue and the gingiva. It treats stiffness of the tongue.

Shen Gen: This point is located in the depression at the root of the frenulum. It treats hypertension and cerebral thrombosis.

Zuo Quan: This point is located near the openings of sublingual glands. It treats the sequelae of cerebral vascular accidents.

Ye Fang: This point is inside sublingual veins near the root of the tongue. It is indicated for hypertension and the sequelae of cerebral vascular accidents.

Zhi Mai: This point is located outside the sublingual veins near the tip of the tongue. It is indicated for hypertension and the sequelae of cerebral vascular accidents.

Choosing tongue acupoints for the treatment of stroke

There are five different methods for choosing acupoints on the tongue for the treatment of stroke. First, one can choose points according to TCM pattern discrimination.

For example, for the treatment of insomnia, one can use Heart, Kidney, and Frontal points. Secondly, one can use what is called inside-outside matching. In this case, one combines tongue points with regular points near the head. For example, for post-stroke tongue stiffness, one can use *Zhong Ju* plus *Lian Quan* (CV 23). Third, there is top-bottom matching. Here, tongue points are combined with points on the conception or governing vessel and the lower limbs. For example, for urgent, rough or choppy urination, and urinary pain, one can use the Bladder tongue point with *Zhong Ju.* The fourth method is called ipsilateral left-right matching. It consists of combining tongue points with points on the four limbs. An example of this type of point selection would be using right Lung and Throat with right *Shao Shang* (LU 11) for right-sided throat pain. The fifth and last method of tongue point selection is called contralateral left-right matching. For example, to treat paralysis or pain of the left upper limb, one can use right Upper Limb and Spleen tongue points matched with left *Qu Chi* (LI 11) and *He Gu* (LI 4). The foregoing ipsilateral and contralateral methods can be used either singly or in combination. For example, to treat facial paralysis, stiffness of

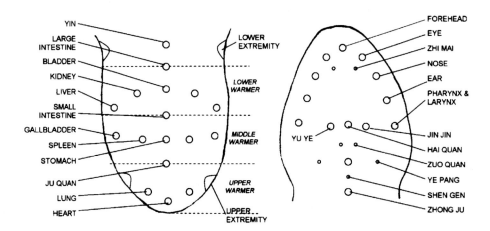

The Top Surface of the Tongue   The Bottom Part of the Tongue

tongue, hemiplegia, a purple tongue, and a tight pulse, the practitioner may use Kidney, Liver, Heart, and *Zhong Ji* (CV 3) combined with *Bai Hui* (GV 20), *Qu Chi* (LI 11), *Lao Gong* (Per 8), *Zu San Li* (St 36), *Zhao Hai* (Ki 6), and *Tai Chong* (Liv 3).

Treatment method[23]

Before the procedure, the patient should gargle with a 3% solution of H_2O_2 or 1/5000 potassium permanganate. The tongue is then held using gauze or, to access the bottom surface, the patient rolls up his or her tongue and it is pressed against the upper teeth. The needle is quickly inserted to a depth of approximately one *fen* and manipulated by both thrusting-lifting and twisting-rotating. For supplementation, a 1-1.5 inch 30 gauge filiform needle is inserted and rotated clockwise 3-9 times. This procedure is repeated 3-9 times as needed. During rotation, the needle may reach a depth of 0.5-1.0 *fen*, although shallow insertion helps reduce the chance of bleeding. For drainage, a 1-1.5 inch 28 gauge filiform needle is used and rotated counterclockwise six times. This procedure was generally repeated six or eight times. With the deeper needle insertion, bleeding becomes a possibility. When using bleeding technique, one-inch 26 gauge needles may be used. Rapid tapping is then done to let 2-3 drops of blood out. Afterwards, patients should gargle with 1/5000 furancillin solution.

When doing tongue acupuncture, there are several precautions which should be observed. First, one should strictly observe sterile procedures. Secondly, be careful about needle insertion depth and technique. Third, if the patient is nervous, have them lie down during the procedure. Fourth, when bleeding, afterwards use a sterile cotton ball with pressure on the point to stop bleeding. Fifth, do not use this method in emergency cases.

Tongue acupuncture indications & contraindications

Tongue acupuncture is indicated for diseases of the tongue, such as deviation, double tongue (sublingual swelling), strange tastes in the mouth, or throat pain as well as paralysis, numbness, or pain of the limbs and torso. Because of its connection to the organs, the tongue can also be effective for treating hypertension, periarthritis, heart, or other visceral diseases. This method is contraindicated if the patient has a tendency to bleed.

Clinical trial[24]

The following study compared tongue acupuncture plus body needles to using only body acupuncture. It involved 156 cases, with 78 patients in both the treatment and comparison groups. Ages and gender were about the same for both groups: 29 patients were younger than 50, 69 cases were between 51-60 years, 40 cases were between ages 61-70, and 18 cases were 71 or older. Of all the cases, 58 were affected on the left side, 97 on the right side, and one person was affected on both sides. Most of the patients had speech difficulties, facial paralysis, and hemiplegia.

Treatment of those in the treatment group consisted of two needles in the base of the neck and tongue points. No tongue or neck needles were used in the comparison group. The main tongue points used in the treatment group were Kidney, Brain, and Sublingual. For ischemia, the sublingual gland inside of the sublingual artery on left and right was added. For hemorrhage, a point approximately five *fen* behind the center point on the top surface of the tongue was added. For speech problems, Heart was added. Needles at the nape of the neck consisted of a point 1.5 inches bilateral to *Ya*

Men (GV 15). These needles were inserted towards the opposite side while taking precautions as this is potentially dangerous.

All members of the comparison group were needled at *Jian Yu* (LI 15), *Qu Chi* (LI 11), *He Gu* (LI 4), *Huan Tiao* (GB 30), *Feng Shi* (GB 31), *Yang Ling Quan* (GB 34), and *Xuan Zhong* (GB 39). For speech difficulties, *Ya Men* (GV 15) and *Feng Fu* (GV 16), and *Lian Quan* (CV 23) were added. For facial paralysis, *Di Cang* (St 4), *Jia Che* (St 6), *Yang Bai* (GB 14), and *Yi Feng* (TB 17) were added. In the comparison group, patients rested on their healthy side, and the main points were connected to a G6805 electro-acupuncture device with the needles retained for 30 minutes.

There were significant differences in outcomes when the two groups were compared. The treatment group had a cure rate of 64.1%, marked effect rate of 21.8%, and a some effect rate of 11.5%. Therefore, the total effectiveness rate was 97.4%. The comparison group only had a total effectiveness rate of 92.7% (P<0.05). The fact that the majority of patients in the treatment group got good results is believed to be due to the tongue's relationship to the heart and spleen. It also is rich in nerve endings and vessels which connect it to the whole body. Through both the brain and the viscera and bowels connection, points on the tongue can regulate, stimulate, and balance organs to transform phlegm, dispel stasis, and clear the mind. The addition of the neck points affects the bladder channel which also goes to the brain. Therefore, the patient gets the benefit of both an external and internal treatment.

Chinese Awn Needle Acupuncture

This is a running needling technique which uses special long, fine, and flexible needles to obtain a stronger sensation to awaken the nervous system. Although the use of awn needle acupuncture is not common, it has recently been used in China to treat patients following stroke. The following two studies show that its efficacy is promising and is obviously better than that of conventional acupuncture. In the first study, 220 patients were diagnosed by cranial CT scan as paralyzed stroke patients in various stages of recovery.[25] Among these, 128 were males and 92 were females. Twelve patients were 40 years old or younger, 80 patients were 41-55 years old, 110 patients were 56-70 years old, and 18 patients were older than 71. In terms of the type of stroke, 131 patients were recovering from cerebral infarction from arterial thrombosis, and 89 patients from hemorrhage. In 102 cases, the infarctions happened in the left cerebrum; in 115 cases, in the right, and in three cases, on both sides. These 220 patients were randomly divided into two groups–120 patients were in the treatment group, another 100 patients were in the comparison group. There was no significant difference between the two groups in age, sex, or disease condition.

All members of the treatment group were needled at *Chuan Zhi*[26] plus five pairs of points using running needle method:

Jian Yu (LI 15) ——————→*Qu Chi* (LI 11)
Pian Li (LI 6) ——————→*Qu Chi* (LI 11)
He Gu (LI 4) ——————→ *Hou Xi* (SI 3)
Bi Guan (St 31) ——————→ *Cheng Fu* (Bl 36)
Feng Long (St 40) ——————→ *Zhu Bin* (Ki 9)

Auxiliary points included:

For facial paralysis:

Di Cang (St 4) ——————→*Jia Che* (St 6)
Ying Xiang (LI 20) →*Yin Tang* (M-HN-3)

For speech difficulties:

Shang Lian Quan (M-HN-21) and *Ju Quan* (M-HN-36)

The patients were asked to lie supine. Then *Chuan Zhi* was inserted with the tip of the needle pointed forward. The insertion was at the side of the spinous process between the second and third cervical vertebra. The depth of insertion was 2-3 inches.[27] The patient should have felt local numbness and distention radiating to the same side of the upper and lower limbs. Once the qi was obtained, the needles were immediately removed. When manipulating the needles, the practitioner produced a sensation that the patient felt radiating as far as possible into their extremities. The needles were retained in the body for 30 minutes.

For *Shang Lian Quan*, a 2.5 inch needle was inserted towards the root of the tongue, using a special needle manipulation technique named *He Gu* needling. [28] The needle was withdrawn immediately after manipulation. As for *Ju Quan*, a 2.5-3 inch needle was inserted from the tongue body to its root. The needle was withdrawn after obtaining the qi. For acupoints on the face, 2-3 inch needles were used with draining hand technique. The needles were retained in the body for 30 minutes and were manipulated once every 10 minutes. Acupuncture was given once per day, with 20 treatments equaling one course.

All members of the comparison group received the following acupuncture. For paralysis in the body, *Jian Yu* (LI 15), *Qu Chi* (LI 11), *He Gu* (LI 4), *Wai Guan* (TB 5), *Huan Tiao* (GB 30), *Yang Ling Quan* (GB 34), *Zu San Li* (St 36), *Jie Xi* (St 41), and *Kun Lun* (Bl 60) were needled. For facial paralysis, *Di Cang* (St 4) and *Jia Che*

(St 6) were needled. For speech difficulties, *Ya Men* (GV 15), *Lian Quan* (CV 23), and *Tong Li* (Ht 5) were needled. One to three inch needles were inserted perpendicularly. No supplementing or draining methods were used. The needles were retained in the body for 30 minutes, with the needles being manipulated once every 10 minutes. Acupuncture was done once per day, with 20 treatments equaling one course.

In the treatment group, 74 cases were basically cured, 72 cases showed marked improvement, 61 cases improved, and 23 cases experienced no effect. The results also indicated that the sooner the patients received treatments, the better the results.

In the second clinical trial, there were 27 stroke patients, 17 males and 10 females.[29] Their ages ranged from 20-70 years, with most between ages 40-60. In terms of disease duration, 16 patients were six months post stroke, eight patients were 6-12 months post stroke, and three patients were within three years of their initial stroke. Twenty-three of these patients were paralyzed, seven had speech problems, and three had eye and/or mouth deviation. Twenty-nine to 30 gauge needles 5-7 inches in length were used to needle the following points once per day:

Da Zhui (GV 14) ———>*Zhi Yang* (GV 9)
Shen Dao (GV11) ———>*Jin Suo* (GV 8)
Ming Men (GV 4)———>*Yao Shu* (GV 2)

Two groups of auxiliary points were alternated every other day. For paralyzed upper limb, group one consisted of:

Jian Yu (LI 15) ———> *Bi Nao* (LI 14)

group two consisted of:

Qu Chi (LI 11) ———> *Shao Hai* (Ht 3)

For paralyzed lower limb, group one included:
Bi Guan (St 31) ————————→*Fu Tu* (St 32)

group two included:

San Yin Jiao (Sp 6) → *Xuan Zhong* (GB 39)

For speech difficulties, *Tong Li* (Ht 5) was added.

For eye and mouth deviation:
Di Cang (St 4) ————————→*Jia Che* (St 6) was added.

After insertion, the needles were manipulated for 1-2 minutes every five minutes. The needles were manipulated three times in total during each treatment session. The level of sensation from the manipulation was whatever the patient could bear. Using this protocol, nine cases (33.3%) were basically cured, eight cases (29.6%) got a marked effect, nine cases (33.3%) improved, and one case (3.8%) got no effect. Therefore, the total effectiveness rate was 96.2%. Awn needle acupuncture is unique in that it uses such long needles, punctures so deeply, and creates such strong needle sensation. Stimulating the governing vessel, it regulates the qi and brightens the spirit. Qi is then able to reach the affected area, and the immune system is stimulated in order to restore bodily functions, harmonize yin and yang, and finally bring back vitality. In some cases, rheoencephalogram was used to observe the immediate effect of awn needle acupuncture. It showed that the hemodynamic had significantly improved after acupuncture and proved the effectiveness of this needling technique of running one needle through several acupoints. Contraindications when needling the governing channel include no deep insertion, no repeated manipulation, and no pulling or thrusting the needles too vigorously. These are to avoid damaging the spinal cord.

Wrist–Ankle Needling Method

This is a simple, safe technique due to its use of superficial needle insertion and few needles. It is also a relatively new technique. Its strengths are safety, convenience, and fast-recovery of the patient. The original clinical application of this method was for mental and neural disorders. Nowadays, its wide clinical use includes the treatment of stroke. In the following clinical trial, there were 15 hemiplegia stroke patients, 11 males and four females.[30] Their ages ranged from 50-65 years. Nine cases were within three months of the onset of their stroke, four cases were from six months to one year, and two cases were from 1-5 years. Ten of these cases were due to cerebral infarction, four cases were due to hemorrhage, and one case was due to subdural hematoma. Symptoms included lack of strength in the extremities, loss of mobility, generalized numbness, and, in the more severe cases, mouth deviation and aphasia.

Wrist points were named "Upper" and ankle points were named "Lower". The wrist points were located two inches above the transverse crease of the wrist. The first wrist point started on the ulnar side of the palmar aspect and continued around to the dorsal aspect. The ankle points were located three inches above the medial and lateral maleolus. The first ankle point started from the medial aspect of the tendon calcaneus. It then continued around to the lateral border of the tendon of the muscle calcaneus. Upper One[31] of the paralyzed side was used to treat body numbness. Upper Five[32] was used to increase grasping strength and the mobile function of the upper limbs. Lower One[33] was used to increase the strength and mobility function of lower extremities, and Lower Six[34] was used to treat difficulty of hip flexion and knee extension.

Four centimeter silver needles were inserted obliquely at a 30 degree angle into the skin. Following the vertical axis of the limb, needles were then moved forward slowly in the subcutaneous tissues. The needles reached a maximum depth of 3.8 centimeters. When the patient no longer had difficulty in hip flexion and knee extension on the affected side, Lower Six was no longer needled. However, when the patient's condition fluctuated, relaying needling technique[35] at Upper Five and Lower One was administered. The needles were manipulated using supplementing or draining techniques in order to increase the efficacy of the treatment by increasing the stimulation of the needles. However, the patients did not need to have the qi sensation from this needling technique. Generally, acupuncture was done once per day and 10 days equaled one course of treatment. Needles were retained in the body for an hour. If the treatment had not reached its desired effect in one course, a second course of treatment was resumed after 5-6 days of rest. Typically, patients needed 4-6 courses of treatment. In general, patients were able to recover completely after three months of treatment and were able to take part in strenuous physical activities. In 10 cases on follow-up, there was no relapse within six months to two years after cessation of treatment.

Normally, after the first few treatments, the patient had some positive responses, such as increased grasping ability in the upper limbs, increased relaxation of the leg muscles, increased hip flexion and knee extension, and decreased numbness. This was often followed by a relapse manifesting as lack of strength of the upper and lower limbs and/or increased numbness. Such relapses usually appeared after 1-2 courses of treatment. In such cases, it was important to continue daily acupuncture during the relapse. After 3-5 more treatments, the patient would usually regain the strength in their upper and lower limbs and experience less numbness and more mobility. The patient's condition typically improved after each relapse. Generally speaking, the greater the severity of the relapse, the faster mobility was subsequently restored along with less numbness. Normally, the patient experienced 3-4 relapses before full recovery. The speed of recovery was fastest when treatment was started within three months of the stroke. Nevertheless, there are several reasons why this treatment may be ineffective. These include initiation of treatment after more than three months delay following a stroke, older age, insensitive nerve endings in the subcutaneous tissues, or lack of cooperation of the patients with the treatment.

Magnetic Acupoint Therapy

Magnetic acupoint therapy consists of using magnets on acupuncture points. This technique combines the benefits of both acupuncture theory and the magnetic field. This method is particularly effective for treating the sequelae of stroke. It helps restore upper extremity function as well as mobility. In addition, it is an exceptionally good treatment method for patients who are afraid of needles. The following are two clinical studies of magnetic acupoint therapy which address these topics. In the first,[36] 62 hospitalized patients were diagnosed by cranial CT scan or MRI as suffering from stroke. These 62 patients were then randomly divided into two groups. Treatment group was treated with magnetic-field plus point stimulation. The comparison group was treated by electro-acupuncture.

Altogether, there were 42 males and 20 females with an average age of 61. In terms of stroke history, 48 patients had experienced their stroke within three months, while 14 patients were 4-6 months out from their stroke. Further, there were 51 cases of cerebral thrombosis and 11 cases of cerebral hemorrhage.

All members of the treatment group were treated with magnets which were 1.3 centimeters in diameter and 0.5cm in thickness with a magnetic field of 3000GS as well as with a multifunction electric pulse point stimulator with 0.6-1.3 Hertz. Either cranial areas or associated diseased areas scanned by CT or MRI were selected for treatment. Only six acupoints from each upper and lower extremity were chosen per treatment. The channels and acupoints selected were based on Brunnstrom"s classification of bodily function.[37] After the magnets were firmly taped on top of the acupoints, the electric pulse point was connected to the magnets. Each treatment lasted 30 minutes and was done once per day. Point selection depended on the stage of the disease. Stage I patients'strokes had occurred from a few days up to two weeks prior to treatment. In these cases, acupoints were mainly chosen from the yang channels. These included *Jian Yu* (LI 15), *Qu Chi* (LI 11), *Shou San Li* (LI 10), *Liang Qiu* (St 34), *Zu San Li* (St 36), and *Yang Ling Quan* (GB 34). Stage II and III patients'strokes had occurred from 2-4 weeks prior to treatment. In these cases, acupoints from both yin and yang channels were chosen, including *Jian Yu* (LI 15), *Qu Chi* (LI 11), *Shou San Li* (LI 10), *Tian Fu* (Lu 3), *Xia Bai* (Lu 4), *Qu Ze* (Per 3), *Xi Men* (Per 4), *Liang Qiu* (St 34), *Zu San Li* (St 36), *Yang Ling Quan* (GB 34), *Yin Ling Quan* (Sp 9), *Xue Hai* (Sp 10), and *Zhao Hai* (Ki 6). Stages IV, V, and VI patients'strokes had occurred over four

weeks prior to treatment. In these cases, acupoints were mainly chosen from the yin channels with some auxiliary points on the yang channels. These points included *Tian Fu* (Lu 3), *Xia Bai* (Lu 4), *Qu Ze* (Per 3), *Xi Men* (Per 4), *Shao Fu* (Ht 8), *Wai Guan* (TB 5), *Shou San Li* (LI 10), *Xue Hai* (Sp 10), *Yin Ling Quan* (Sp 9), *San Yin Jiao* (Sp 6), *Zhao Hai* (Ki 6), *Liang Qiu* (St 34), and *Zu San Li* (St 36).

All members of the comparison group received electro-acupuncture with a continuous frequency of 0.6-1.3 Hertz using a G6805-I electro-acupuncture device. The main acupoints used were chosen from the yang ming channels coupled with some points from the tai yang and shao yang. These included *Jian Yu* (LI 15), *Qu Chi* (LI 11), *Shou San Li* (LI 10), *He Gu* (LI 4), *Wai Guan* (TB 5), *Huan Tiao* (GB 30), *Yang Ling Chuan* (GB 34), *Zu San Li* (St 36), *Jie Xi* (St 41), and *Kun Lun* (Bl 60). Cranial acupoints consisted of Motor Area and Leg Motor and Sensory Area. Qi was obtained after needling, and electrical stimulation was applied for 30 minutes per treatment once per day.

Both the treatment and the comparison groups showed improvement as far as restoring the function of the upper extremities and walking abilities were concerned. The total effectiveness rates were 93.35% in the treatment group and 70.09% on the comparison group (P> 0.05). Thus, it was clear that those in the treatment group achieved better results.

In the second clinical trial using magnet acupoint therapy, there were a total of 232 patients.[38] These patients were randomly divided into two groups of 116 patients–a treatment and a comparison group. In the treatment group, 67 patients were male and

49 were female. The average age in this group was 64. In terms of clinical symptoms, 68 of these patients had paralysis on the left side of the body, while 52 had paralysis on the right. Thirty-eight patients suffered from facial paralysis, 47 patients had speech difficulties, 23 patients suffered from urinary incontinence, and 28 patients had difficulty swallowing. Age, gender, and disease condition was statistically comparable in the comparison group.

In the treatment group, acupuncture needles 0.5-2 inches were first inserted and then magnetic chips (3-4 millimeters in diameter, 1-2 millimeters in thickness, 1600-2000 Gauss with either circular or square shape) were taped on the exposed body of the needles. Treatment was administered once per day for 30 minutes each time, with 10 treatments equaling one course. Patients were then given five days of rest between each successive course. The largest number of courses was four and the shortest was one. Points selected for treatment included the upper 1/5, middle 2/5 of cranial Motor Area or three temporal scalp needles plus *Jian Yu* (LI 15), *Qu Chi* (LI 11), *Shou San Li* (LI 10), *He Gu* (LI 4), *Nei Guan* (Per 6), and *Wai Guan* (TB 5). If the lower extremities were affected, *Huan Tiao* (GB 30), *Yang Ling Quan* (GB 34), *Fu Tu* (St 32), *Zu San Li* (St 36), *Feng Long* (St 40), *Jie Xi* (St 41), *Yin Ling Quan* (Sp 9), and *San Yin Jiao* (Sp 6) were treated. If there was facial paralysis, the lower 2/5 of the cranial Motor Area was treated plus *Quan Liao* (SI 18), *Di Cang* (St 4), *Jia Che* (St 6), and *Ying Xiang* (LI 20). For urinary incontinence or retention, *Qi Hai* (CV 6), *Guan Yuan* (CV 4), *Zhong Ji* (CV 3), *Zhong Shu* (GV 7), *Shen Shu* (Bl 23), and *Pang Guang Shu* (Bl 28) were treated. For speech difficulties, cranial Motor Speech Area was treated along with *Lian Quan* (CV 23). Regular

acupuncture was performed at the same acupoints on all the patients in the comparison group.

Both the treatment and comparison groups showed improvements in terms of their ability to walk (with or without assistance) and the disappearance of associated symptoms. The total effectiveness rates were 85.34% and 68.96% respectively for the treatment and comparison groups ($P < 0.01$).

When a magnet of 1600-2000 Gauss is taped onto a one inch long needle, the tip of the needle will receive 1/10 of the magnetic effect (*i.e.*, 160-200 Gauss), while a two inch needle will receive 1/20 of the magnetic effect (*i.e.*, 80-100 Gauss). When the magnetic acupoint therapy is administered on, for example, *Wai Guan* (TB 5), the amount of magnetism can be measured on *Nei Guan* (Per 6). In other words, the magnetic field will pass through both acupoints and hence affect both areas. When magnetic acupuncture was administered only on the cranial area, quite a few patients reported that they felt a warm sensation in their heads. Some patients also reported that they felt fluid moving inside their heads. Magnetic acupuncture therapy is believed to regulate the qi and blood as well as free the flow of the channels and vessels. On the other hand, a magnetic field also affects the movements and conditions of biological molecules. Hence, it will locally or systemically regulate changes in the cells. The combination of magnetic field therapy and acupuncture increases its effectiveness.

Crowded Needling Technique[39]

In this study, 15 needles were inserted closely together on the back of the neck. The benefit of this technique is its strong stimulation. Crowded needling technique was developed from *Nei Jing (Inner Classic)* where it is mentioned in the chapter of the *Ling Shu (Spiritual Axis)* titled "Official Needling." There were 82 patients who suffered from various sequelae ddue to stroke. Among them, 48 cases (58.6%) were cerebral thrombosis, 20 cases (24.4%) were cerebral hemorrhage and 14 cases (17%) were cerebral infarction. According to Wah Yan-ling, patients were treated sitting up in a chair with his or her forehead resting at a downward angle on a pillow on a desk. The three acupoints selected along the governing channel were *Feng Fu* (GV 16), *Ya Men* (GV 15), and *Nao Hu* (GV 17). The neck was then divided into six equal portions from *Wan Gu* (GB 12) to *Feng Fu* (GV 16) bilaterally on a horizontal line. One acupoint was assigned for each equal portion for a total of 15 acupoints.[40] One and a half inch, 28 or 30 gauge, stainless steel needles were inserted perpendicularly into all the acu-

points except *Nao Hu* at which the point of the needle was pointed obliquely downward. The depth of insertion was approximately one inch.[41] Using slight manipulation, the needles were mildly pulled and thrust so the patient felt a distended sensation.[42] The needles were retained for 20-30 minutes per treatment.The treatment was administered once every 1-3 days. Ten treatments equaled one course which followed a week of rest. ANother course of treatments resumed after the rest. The total effectiveness rate was 96.3% with 25.6% cured, 43.9% having a great effect, 26.8% improved and 3.7% with no effect.

The acupoints used in crowded needling technique are situated on the governing vessel and the bladder and gallbladder channels. According to the authors of the *Ling Shu (Spiritual Axis)*, the bladder channel begins at the inner canthus of the eye at *Jing Ming* (Bl 1) and ascends along the forehead to the vertex. From the vertex, one branch enters the brain and meets the governing vessel. The governing vessel starts in the lower abdomen and then runs posteriorly along the midline of the sacrum and the interior of the spinal column to *Feng Fu* (GV 16) where it enters the brain. Clinically, this technique has been used not only for the treatment of post-stroke sequelae, epilepsy and migraine but also for hypertension, allergic asthma, chronic sinusitis, insomnia, and colds.

The Crowded Needling Location

Setting the Mountain on Fire Technique[43]

This supplementing method

generates a warm sensation which enhances the circulation of qi and blood in the affected area, thus facilitating the restoration of bodily functions. The following is a study of using the setting the mountain on fire technique to treat bodily dysfunction due to stroke. All the patients in this clinical trial were diagnosed by CT scan as having suffered a stroke. Both the treatment and comparison groups had 49 patients apiece. The treatment group consisted of 30 males and 19 females. Their ages ranged from 41-90 years. The shortest time since the onset of stroke was nine days and the longest was three years. In terms of type of stroke, 12 subjects had cranial hemorrhage, while 37 subjects had cranial infarction. In the comparison group, 33 were males and 16 were females whose ages ranged from 42-79 years. The shortest time since onset of stroke was nine days and the longest was three years. In terms of type of stroke, 13 of these patients had cranial hemorrhage, while 36 had cranial infarction. All subjects from both groups were also administered a Chinese herbal formula, *Bu Yang Huan Wu Tang* (Supplement Yang & Return Five [Tenths] Decoction).[44]

All members of the treatment group received acupuncture on the affected side of the body at the main points *Ji Quan* (Ht 1) and *Yong Quan* (Ki 1). Then the auxiliary points included *Chi Ze* (Lu 5), *Qu Chi* (LI 11), *Xue Hai* (Sp 10), *Zu San Li* (St 36), and *San Yin Jiao* (Sp 6). Additionally, running needle technique was performed from *He Gu* (LI 4) to *Lao Gong* (Per 8). Twenty-eight gauge, 1.5-2.0 inch long, stainless steel needles were used at each of the above points. Then setting the mountain on fire technique was performed. This technique consisted of inserting the needles successively from shallow (the upper 1/3 level of the acupoint), to middle (the middle 1/3

level) to deep (the lower 1/3 level) levels. At the shallow level, the needles were thrust heavily and then slowly lifted up nine times. This needle manipulation was then repeated at both the middle and deep levels. Finally, the needles were withdrawn to the shallow level. This constituted one cycle, and this cycle was performed three times. Then the needles were retained in the body for 20 minutes. The practitioner mentally focused on the tip of the needle during the insertion, while the subject was instructed to concentrate on the acupoints being needled. The treatment required that the patient experience warm sensation at each of the acupoints. Acupuncture was administered once per day, with five treatments equaling one course. Two days of rest were allowed between each successive course of treatment. All members of the comparison group were needled at the same points as the treatment group. However, neither supplementing nor draining technique was used at any of these points. Treatment duration and frequency were the same as above. Although there was no significant statistical difference between the two groups before treatment (P>0.05), after treatment, there was (P<0.01). The total effectiveness rates in the treatment and comparison groups were 96% and 90% respectively.

According to the authors of this study, regardless of the cause, the disease mechanisms of strokes are stasis and stagnation in the channels and network vessels, non-smooth flow of the qi and blood, and lack of nourishment of the sinews. Setting the mountain on fire technique is one of the eight methods mentioned in the *Jin Zhen Fu (Prose-plus-poem of the Golden Needle)*. It is a warming method which adds yang qi internally so that the subjects would feel warm either locally or throughout the whole body. The resultant abundance of qi under the needles in the channels enhances the circulation of qi and blood. This allows the channels to flow freely, dispersing stagnation, and allowing the sinews and muscles to obtain proper nourishment. As a result, bodily function can be restored. Modern Western medicine believes that bodily dysfunction after a stroke is due to reduced excitability of the nerves which control the motor function. Setting the mountain on fire technique is a strong stimulation method which stimulates the nerves and rebuilds the conditioned reflexes. As the above outcomes show, this method achieves better results than one which uses neither supplementation nor drainage. In general, there is a positive correlation between obtaining the qi and therapeutic effectiveness with acupuncture. As most of the above studies have also shown, the shorter the time since the onset of the illness, the higher the effectiveness rate was and the fewer treatments needed.

Biological Tide of the Flow of Qi & Blood Technique[45]

The following method is one of several based on the timing of the flow of the qi and blood through the body. Its strong points are that it uses few points, is easy to perform, and shows a higher success rate than regular acupuncture. Among the 63 patients enrolled in this study, 53 were male and 10 were female. These patients had an average age of 61.5 years. Diagnosis was made by cranial CT scan followed by TCM pattern discrimination diagnosis. The duration of illness since the onset of stroke ranged from 28-120 days. These 63 patients were randomly divided into two groups–a treatment group of 31patients and a comparison group of 32 patients.

All the patients in this study were treated with acupuncture on the day following hospital admittance. Those in the treatment group were treated with acupuncture using the *fei teng ba fa*. This translates as the flying and soaring eight [points] method. This method uses the eight meeting points of the eight extraordinary vessels. Points were selected by looking up the starting times for *Hou Xi* (SI 3)/*Shen Mai* (Bl 62) on hand and foot *tai yang* channels or *Zu Lin Qi* (GB 41)/*Wai Guan* (TB 5) on the hand and foot shao yang channels in *The Quick Reference Flying & Soaring Eight Methods Time Table*.[46] One or two acupoints were needled daily at a specific time based on the host-guest principle. *Lie Que* (Lu 7) and *Zhao Hai* (Ki 6) were added for those who had speech difficulties. Patients received acupuncture once per day, with the needles being retained for 30 minutes each time. The needles were manipulated with supplementing hand technique. A series of 10 treatments was regarded as one course of treatment, and there was no break between successive courses. Patients were re-evaluated after three courses.

Regular acupuncture was performed on the patients in the comparison group. Acupoints were selected based on the book *Zhen Jiu Xue (The Study of Acupuncture & Moxibustion)*.[47] On the upper limb, the points selected consisted of *Jian Yu* (LI 15), *Qu Chi* (LI 11), *Shou San Li* (LI 10), *Wai Guan* (TB 5), and *He Gu* (LI 4). On the lower limb, the points selected consisted of *Huan Tiao* (GB 30), *Yang Ling Quan* (GB 34), *Zu San Li* (St 36), *Jie Xi* (St 41), and *Kun Lun* (Bl 60). The frequency of treatments and technique were the same as the treatment group.

Results were compared between the two groups in terms of clinical effects on ischemic stroke as well as the change of the indices of nail fold microcirculation[48] and hemorheology.[49] In the treatment group, the basic cure rate was 32.26% and the total effectiveness rate was 93.55%. In the comparison group, the basic cure rate was 21.88% and the total effectiveness rate was 93.75%. Thus there was no significant difference between the two groups in terms of the rate of effectiveness. However, there was a great difference between the groups in terms of cure rates. The indices of nail fold microcirculation and the hemorheology were noticeably improved in both groups. In terms of TCM pattern discrimination, therapeutic efficacy in both groups was higher for those presenting either qi vacuity or phlegm obstruction followed by those presenting yin vacuity. Effectiveness was the least for those presenting internal stirring of liver wind.

Flying and soaring eight [points] method is derived from the principle that qi and blood converge from the 12 regular meridians in the eight extraordinary vessels and that each of these vessels is at high tide at a particular time of each day. It is believed that this technique treats both the root causes and branch or tip manifestation of disease. Since this technique is administered during the time when qi and blood flow converge to the maximum, it boosts the qi and nourishes yin. The technique also quickens the blood and dispels stasis as well as regulates imbalances of yin and yang. Since it only used one or two points located on the extremities, it is also easier to perform than regular acupuncture.

Moxibustion Method[50]

The use of the warming effect of moxibustion to increase the flow of blood in blocked channels is a simple and safe way to treat patients suffering from the effects of stroke. The following protocol has been used by

Zhang Deng-bu for over two decades. He calls his technique the moxibustion method for warming and coursing. Dr. Zhang obtained satisfactory results in treating 38 cases of coronary heart disease and 110 cases of cerebrovascular disease with this method. For angina pectoris and chest qi impediment, Dr. Zhang moxaed *Nei Guan* (Per 6), *Shan Zhong* (CV 17), and *Xin Shu* (Bl 15). For stroke, aphasia, and hemiplegia, he moxaed *Bai Hui* (GV 20) and *Tian Chuang* (SI 16). Moxibustion was done with either supplementation or drainage technique according to the patient's condition. For supplementation, he allowed the fire to extinguish itself. For draining, he extinguished the fire rapidly. Dr. Zhang used mild moxibustion if most of the symptoms were due to a root vacuity even though there was repletion on a superficial level. He held the cones approximately two fingers above the skin of the reclining patient. He first applied moxa bilaterally to *Xin Shu*. Then he turned the patient over and warmed *Nei Guan* and *Shan Zhong* for 5-10 minutes each. For dizziness and insomnia, he added *Shen Men* (Ht 7) and *Zu San Li* (St 36). For hypertension, he added *Bai Hui* (GV 20) and *Tai Chong* (Liv 3). For stroke and hemiplegia, he added *Tian Chuang* on the healthy side first for 15 minutes, then *Bai Hui* (GV 20) for 15 minutes. This treatment was administered 1-2 times per day. For hypertension, he might also include moxibustion at *Tai Xi* (Ki 3) and *Tai Chong* for five minutes on each point. In the two representative cases described in the article, the patients received moxibustion twice a day for five minutes on each selected point, with six treatments equaling one course of treatment. After three to five courses, both patients felt marked improvement. The first case required six courses for a complete cure, while the second case received a total of eight courses before all symptoms disappeared.

According to traditional Chinese medicine, the heart, kidneys, liver, and spleen are involved in coronary heart disease with angina pectoris and chest qi impediment. Both the yang of the kidneys and heart are involved in the creation and control of the yang qi of the body. Typically as we age, yang qi declines. Therefore, blood circulation slows enough to cause heart channel obstruction and pain. Angina pain from yang qi obstruction and blockage can also occur from phlegm ascending from the middle burner, emotions such as anxiety or irritation, or blood vacuity causing malnourishment of the network vessels of the heart. Other factors may also contribute to the symptoms of hemiplegia and aphasia found in stroke victims. These can include liver-kidney yin vacuity, heart fire effulgence, wind phlegm blockage and obstruction, qi stagnation, and/or blood stasis. Although they are different diseases, angina pectoris, stroke, and hemiplegia all result from blood stasis and phlegm obstruction in the channels and network vessels. Thus it follows that warming the channels is an effective treatment. In fact, moxibustion helps to thin the blood and reduce blood pressure, improves blood viscosity and dilates the vessels.

Symmetrical Needling Method[51]

The concept of symmetry, of arranging or balancing the parts of a whole in respect to size, shape, and position on opposite sides of an axis, is a common theme in the practice of acupuncture. The following article shows how the use of symmetry in needling increases the effectiveness of acupuncture in the treatment of stroke. In this clinical trial of 210 cases, there were 118 males 44-78 years of age and 92 females 49-70 years of age. One hundred seven of the males were affected on the left side and 11 on the right

side. In the females, 90 were affected on the right side, while only two were affected on the left side. In 168 of these patients, the complications of stroke included speech disorders, deviation of the mouth, central facial paralysis, and zero degree of muscular tension in the affected limbs. The course of disease ranged from only four days (the patient could walk with the aid of a stick) to three months. Treatments ran from six days to four full courses of 28 days.

Points selected on the upper limb of the healthy side included *Jian Liao* (TB 14), *Jian Yu* (LI 15), *Jian Nei Ling* (M-UE-48), *Qu Chi* (LI 11), *Shou San Li* (LI 10), *Wai Guan* (TB 5), and *He Gu* (LI 4). On the lower limb of the healthy side, *Huan Tiao* (GB 30), *Feng Shi* (GB 31), *Yang Ling Quan* (GB 34), *Zu San Li* (St 36), *Xuan Zhong* (GB 38), *Jie Xi* (St 41), and *Kun Lun* (Bl 60) were needled. For speech disorders and deviation of mouth, *Cheng Jiang* (CV 24), *Di Cang* (St 4), *Tong Li* (Ht 5), and *Jia Che* (St 6) were needled. For acute stroke, the practitioner used draining technique. If the disease was chronic, they applied supplementation method. After arrival of the qi, the needles were retained for 30 minutes. The points on the healthy side of the body were needled continuously for three treatments. Points chosen on the affected side varied with the sex of the client. For male patients, the same points were selected on both the upper and lower limbs. For female patients, *San Yin Jiao* (Sp 6) was added, retaining the needles for one hour. The points on the affected side were needled once every other day.

In this study, cure was defined as a return to normal of the functions of the affected limbs with the patient able to return to normal life with clear speech and normal thinking. A marked effect was defined as basic recovery of limb function. The patient was able to manage his or her daily life activities with an effort and exhibited normal thinking and speech. Improved meant that improvement of signs and symptoms was markedly obvious. Some progress meant that the paralyzed limb could be bent and stretched out. However, problems with speech still existed. No effect meant that there was no improvement after treatment. Based on these criteria, 120 of the 210 cases treated were cured, 50 obtained a marked effect, 32 improved, five cases showed some progress, and three cases exhibited no effect. Thus the total effectiveness rate was 98.5%.

Acupuncture has already been proven to clear and free the flow of the channels and network vessels, invigorate the body's metabolism and immune system, and improve the circulation of blood. To improve the results in the treatment of stroke, the authors found that first needling on the healthy side strengthens the circulation of qi and blood. That, in turn, increases the nourishment of the tissues and helps rebalance the internal organs. This technique is also less stressful to the affected side and, potentially, offers a shorter and more effective course of treatment.

Herbal Patch Application Method[52]

The herbal patch application method consists of placing herbal plaster over specific acupoints, thus gaining the effects of the Chinese medicinals and channel and network vessels theory. This is a painless, sanitary, and convenient method which does not produce blisters or scars on the skin. In the following study, there was a treatment group of 228 patients consisting of 107 males and 121 females. These patients' ages ranged from 40-76 years. The shortest dura-

tion of illness from the onset of stroke was two days and the longest was 15 years. In terms of TCM pattern discrimination, 164 cases presented with stroke of channels and network vessels and 64 cases presented with stroke of viscera and bowels. In addition, six cases were predicted by stroke reports, 62 cases were examined by CT scan., and 62 cases had their blood lipids compared before and after treatment. There was also a comparison group of another 70 patients. Of these, 26 were male and 44 were female. These patients' ages ranged from 40-75 years. The shortest duration of illness from onset of stroke was three days and the longest was two years. In terms of TCM pattern discrimination, 48 cases were classified as stroke of the channels and network vessels and 22 as stroke of the viscera and bowels.

All members of the treatment group were treated by the application of herbal plasters to various acupoints. The Chinese medicinals used in these patches or plasters were modified according to the individual patient's pattern discrimination. However, the main ingredients included *Quan Xie* (Scorpio), *Dan Shen* (Radix Salviae Miltiorrhizae), *Yan Hu Suo* (Rhizoma Corydalis), and *Dan Pi* (Cortex Moutan). The powdered medicinals were prepared into a disk-shaped paste with a diameter of 16mm. The paste was applied to an adhesive backing and sealed for storage and eventual use. These plasters were applied to *Lian Quan* (CV 23), *Hua Gai* (CV 20), *Shen Que* (CV 8), and bilaterally to *Yong Quan* (Ki 1). However, the selection of acupoints was also modified according to the patient's pattern discrimination. The plasters were changed once per day, with 15 days equaling one course of treatment. After 2-4 courses of treatment, outcomes were evaluated.

Although acupuncture was administered to all members of the comparison group on the three hand and feet yang channels, the main focus was on the yang ming channels. On the upper limbs, the points needled included *Jian Yu* (LI 15), *Qu Chi* (LI 11), *He Gu* (LI 4), and *Wai Guan* (TB 5). On the lower limbs, the points needled were *Zu San Li* (St 36), *Yang Ling Quan* (GB 34), and *Xuan Zhong* (GB 39). Modifications were also made according to the patient's pattern discrimination. Acupuncture was performed once per day, with 30 treatments equaling one course. Outcomes were analyzed after 2-4 courses of treatment.

The total effectiveness rates in the treatment and comparison groups were 92.11% and 88.57% respectively. In the treatment group, 44 of the 62 patients who had their blood lipids examined before treatment had normal cholesterol levels and 38 patients had normal triglyceride levels. After treatment, all the patients returned to normal levels.

The lungs govern the qi and are the florid canopy which face the hundreds of vessels. Therefore, *Hua Gai* (*i.e.,* Florid Canopy) from the conception vessel was selected to free the flow of the qi and blood and regulate the viscera and bowels. *Lian Quan* is a main point for treating loss of voice after stroke and for facial paralysis. *Shen Que* is a root of life. All three acupoints are located on the conception vessel which is the meeting of yin channels. The circulation of the 12 regular channels starts from the conception and governing vessels. *Yong Quan* is the well point on the kidney channel, and well points are points where yin and yang interchange. Thus this point regulates yin and yang as well as strengthens the sinews and bones. Further, it is said that,

To treat wind, treat the blood first. When

the blood moves, wind is automatically extinguished.

It is also said,

If the qi moves, the blood moves. If the qi stops, the blood stops.

Therefore, the main ingredients in the above herbal patches were medicinals that move qi, quicken the blood and transform stasis, dispel wind and free the flow of the network vessels. Herbal patches can strongly boost the qi, strengthen the sinews, free the flow of the vessels, warm the channels, and dispel cold in addition to quickening the blood and stopping pain. They can be used to prevent and treat the aftereffects of stroke.

Acupoint Hot Compress Method[53]

This method, which consists of the application of warm herbal pads on acupoints, is also a needle-free treatment and is both painless and safe. It is suitable for any TCM type of wind stroke patient and good for the patient who is afraid of needles. In the following study, all 323 patients were diagnosed by CT scan as having suffered a stroke. They had been hospitalized within the first week of September, 1997. All were first-time stroke victims. The subjects were randomly divided into a treatment and a comparison group. In the treatment group, there were 128 males and 79 females whose ages ranged from 48-75 years. The patients in the treatment group were further subdivided into five groups according to TCM pattern discrimination. Twenty-seven cases presented with ascendant liver yang hyperactivity; 46 presented with wind phlegm blocking the network vessels; 22 presented with visceral heat phlegm repletion; 58 presented with qi vacuity and blood stasis; and 54 presented with yin vacuity causing internal wind. In the comparison group, there were 68 males and 48 females whose ages ranged from 46-78 years. There were no significant differences in terms of sex, age, or distribution and muscular strength in affected limbs between the two groups (P>0.05). Both the treatment and comparison groups received standard Western medical care from neurologists. The treatment group also received the hot rubbing method at certain acupoints. Most of the acupoints were chosen from the hand and foot yang channels. Acupoints on the affected upper limbs included *He Gu* (LI 4), *Wai Guan* (TB 5), *Shou San Li* (LI 10), *Qu Chi* (LI 11), and *Jian Yu* (LI 15). Acupoints on the affected lower limbs included *Huan Tiao* (GB 30), *Wei Zhong* (Bl 40), *Zu San Li* (St 36), and *Jie Xi* (St 41). According to the condition of paralysis, 3-4 acupoints were chosen each time. Several hot-compress herbal bags were fully soaked in an appropriate volume of water. Then the herbal bags and the water were heated. When they started to boil, the fire was turned to medium/low for 10 minutes. One herbal bag was removed from the herbal liquid and wrapped and kept warm in a towel which had been soaked with the herbal liquid. An acupoint on the affected side was first tapped lightly with the herbal towel until the skin turned red and warm. Then the herbal bag was placed on the acupoint for 20 minutes. Both upper and lower limbs were treated with the hot compress method once per day. One month of treatment was regarded as one course. Each herbal bag was used 1-2 times. To avoid burns during treatment, the temperature of the herbal liquid and bags was carefully monitored. Too low a temperature could also affect the treatment's effectiveness. Subjects were kept warm to avoid catching a cold. On the second day of hospitalization, all subjects had six milliliters of fasting venous blood drawn. Tests for blood rheology, especially total blood viscosity and hematocrit were done. In addition, clinical signs and symptoms, the muscular strength of affected limbs, the patient's walking ability, and changes in the patient's tongue and pulse were observed. The total effectiveness rates in the treatment and comparison groups were 89.86% and 75.00% respectively (P<0.01). There was no significant difference in effectiveness within the treatment group among the different TCM patterns (P>0.05). This demonstrates that the hot compress method is suitable for any TCM pattern of stroke. The total blood viscosity and hematocrit were both elevated before treatment (P>0.05), and there was no significant difference in these between the treatment and comparison groups. After treatment, there was a significant difference in total viscosity and hematocrit between the two groups (P<0.01). This demonstrates that the treatment received by the treatment group was more effective in lowering both total blood viscosity and hematocrit than that received by the comparison group.

According to the authors of this study, the disease mechanisms of wind stroke can be divided into vacuity (root) and repletion (branch or tip). The vacuity mechanisms include liver-kidney yin depletion and qi and blood vacuity. The repletion mechanism include wind yang, liver fire, phlegm heat, and blood stasis. Blockage in the channels results when wind, fire, phlegm, and/or stasis pass through the channels and network vessels. Once the qi and blood have become stagnant, the body lacks nourishment and this leads to paralysis. Although vacuity is involved in the acute stage, repletion is the main manifestation which should be treated first. The objective of treatment at this stage should be to quicken the blood, transform the stasis, and free the flow of the channels.

The herbal bags were prepared by the authors' hospital. The medicinal ingredients included *Kuan Jin Teng* (Radix Tinosporae Sinensis), *Xu Duan* (Radix Dipsaci), etc. Each bag weighed 150 grams. The herbs had the functions of moving the qi, quickening the blood, transforming stasis, and, at the same time, supplementing the liver and kidneys. By applying the hot compress method on acupoints, the herbs reacted directly with the channels and network vessels. As a result, the channels were disinhibited, qi stagnation was dispersed, and blood stasis was dispelled. Since the flow of qi and blood was freed, the affected areas were able to obtain proper nourishment and the goal of treatment was achieved.

Yang governs movement. Therefore, the inability of the body to move is a disease associated with yang. Thus, acupoints from the three hand and foot yang channels were chosen. Since the yang ming channel has lots of qi and lots of blood, it is easier to restore the bodily movement function by freeing the flow of this channel and its abundant righteous qi. According to the channel pathways of the upper and lower limbs, acupoints from the three yang were administered with the purpose to disinhibit both the three yang channels and network vessels and to regulate and rectify the qi and blood. By so doing, the sinews and muscles were nourished, enhancing recovery.

Hot compresses belong to external medicine. In his book, Wu Shang, a famous Chinese doctor in the Qing dynasty, mentioned that hot treatment was the best external treatment. Hot treatment can be applied in both vacuity and repletion cases. The functions of the medicinals in the hot compress method is to quicken blood and transform stasis. This is an attacking and draining method. However, although all wind stroke patients have a root of vacuity, the hot compress method does not aggravate the vacuity condition. Clinically, repletion cases like phlegm heat and ascendant liver yang hyperactivity respond well to the hot compress method as well, and symptoms of heat are not aggravated. From the analysis of blood rheology, the hot compress method lowered the total blood viscosity and the hematocrit. It is speculated that the treatment speeded up the circulation of blood and that the aggregation of the red blood cells was inhibited. Clinically, it was observed that the hot compress method also improved numbness in the affected limbs, joint pain, and any local edema.

He Gu Needling Method[54]

This is a special insertion technique which uses either one needle or three needles. When one needle is used, it is first inserted perpendicularly downward, then withdrawn upward and inserted to one side and then the same to the other side without the needle being removed from the skin. When three needles are used, one needle is inserted perpendicularly downward and then one needle each angled to the left and right entering the skin at the same point. This technique is used in areas with relatively thick muscles. It is one of the five ancient needling methods mentioned in the chapter "Official Needling" in the *Ling Shu (Spiritual Pivot)*. In the following study, this method was used to treat 215 stroke patients. All 215 patients were diagnosed as having apoplectic hemiplegia by CT scan. Among these, 135 were male and 80 were female. The youngest age was 39 years old and the oldest was 85 years of age. All the patients were in the recovery stages. One hundred eighty-four had suffered a stroke within a month of the beginning of the study, while 31 had suffered their stroke more than a month before beginning the study. One hundred thirty-two had cerebral infarction, 79 had cerebral hemorrhage, and four had a mixed diagnosis. These 215 patients were randomly divided into two groups–a treatment group of 108 patients treated with *He Gu* needling and a comparison group of 107 patients treated Western medicine.

Acupuncture was administered to all members of the treatment group on the affected side of the body. Two to three inch needles were inserted at *Shou San Li* (LI 10) and *Fu Tu* (St 32) with the *He Gu* needling technique. The needle was inserted obliquely towards the medial side of the arm and leg approximately 1.5-2.5 inches at both points. The needles were lifted and thrust repeatedly for a minute without using either supplementing or draining hand technique. At the same acupoints the procedure was repeated and the needles were lifted up under the skin to change their direction towards the lateral side with an oblique insertion. Finally, the direction of the needles was changed a third time to point obliquely along the flow of the yang ming channel. This treatment was regarded as more effective when spasm of the fingers or toes was observed during the needle manipulation. The needles were retained for 20 minutes each treatment and were manipulated once midway during the retention. Acupuncture was administered once per day. Outcomes were analyzed after 20 such treatments. All the patients in the comparison group were treated with standard Western medication and applied hyperbaric oxygen.

Outcomes of this study were graded using six levels.[55] The markedly effective rate and the total effectiveness rates were 66.7% and 91.7% respectively in the treatment group,

while these rates were 29.0% and 77.6% respectively in the comparison group.[56] This difference between the treatment and comparison groups was considered statistically significant ($P < 0.01$).

According to Dr. Liu, the yang ming channel has lots of qi and lots of blood which nourish the congenital sinews that benefit the joints. After a stroke, the qi is stagnant and the blood is static, and the sinews are not properly nourished, thus resulting in reduced physical ability. The purpose of using *Shou San Li* and *Fu Tu* with the *He Gu* needling technique was to stimulate the qi in the yang ming channels, resulting in the smooth flow of qi and blood to the atrophic part of the body. As a result, the sinews were nourished and the function of the paralyzed body was restored. From the biomedical point of view, apoplectic hemiplegia is due to the paralysis of upper motor neurons. The lower motor neurons, which control the muscles, are intact. Although the paralyzed muscles cannot be moved voluntarily, a somatic reflex can be induced by stimulating the reflex center of the spinal cord. Since *Shou San Li* and *Fu Tu* lie in the thick muscles, needling both points with the *He Gu* needling technique affects the flexors and extensors of the forearm and the quadriceps femoris of the lower limb. The flexors and extensors of the forearm control the flexion and extension of the joint at the elbow and wrist. The quadriceps femoris controls the extension of the leg and the flexion of the thigh. As a result, the above acupuncture technique causes the paralyzed muscles to contract automatically. Therefore, muscular atrophy can be prevented. In addition, through repeated stimulation of the peripheral receptors, the brain cells were stimulated, resulting in the restoration of the normal reflex arc.

Extraordinary Electro-acupuncture Plus Moxibustion[57]

In this study, the application of electro-acupuncture on the scalp was combined with direct moxibustion in the treatment of the sequelae of stroke. The conditions treated in this trial included apoplectic hemiplegia, sensory disturbance of the skin, numb extremities, cold body temperature, speech difficulties, and unilateral flaccidity or rigidity. Altogether, there were 204 patients enrolled in this two-wing comparative trial who were diagnosed as having had strokes. One hundred thirteen of these were male and 91 were female. The youngest subject was 38 and the oldest was 86 years old. The average age was 62 years old. These 204 patients were randomly divided into two groups of 102 patients each—a treatment group and a comparison group. The occurrence of the strokes ranged from as recent as two days to six years prior to treatment. Among the subjects, 131 had cerebral infarction and 73 had cerebral hemorrhage. In terms of symptoms, 116 had left paralysis and 88 had right paralysis. Seventeen experienced speech difficulties and 109 had deviation of the mouth. Outcomes between the two groups were analyzed after three months of treatment.

In the treatment group, acupuncture was performed using running needle technique from *Bai Hui* (GV 20) to *Qu Bin* (GB 7) along with electrical stimulation. In other words, a 0.35mm x 40mm needle was inserted at *Bai Hui* through the skin to the subcutaneous layers and pointed in the direction of *Qu Bin*. The needle was inserted in three phases followed by quick manipulation. A G6805 electro-acupuncture machine was used at a frequency of 3.5 Hertz.

Acupuncture was performed on the above scalp areas once per day, with 10 treatments equaling one course of therapy. Three to five days of rest were allowed between each successive course of treatment. In addition, the following scalp acupuncture areas were needled without electrical stimulation: A) Motor and Sensory Area of the Foot and B) First, Second and Third Speech Areas. If there was upper limb paralysis, the 12 well points were bled and *Feng Chi* (GB 20), *Jian Zhen* (SI 9), *Qu Chi* (LI 11), *Shou San Li* (LI 10), *Wai Guan* (TB 5), and *He Gu* (LI 4) were needled. If there was lower limb paralysis, *Shen Shu* (Bl 23), *Huan Tiao* (GB 30), *Bi Guan* (St 31), *Yang Ling Quan* (GB 34), *San Yin Jiao* (Sp 6), *Xuan Zhong* (GB 39), *Jie Xi* (St 41), *Tai Xi* (Ki 3), and *Tai Chong* (Liv 3) were needled. If there was difficulty swallowing, *Lian Quan* (CV 23) was added. For aphasia, *Jin Jin & Yu Ye* (M-HN-20) were bled once every 3-5 days. For speech difficulties, *Lian Quan* (CV 23) and *Tong Li* (Ht 5) were added. For deviation of the mouth, *Di Cang* (St 4), *Qian Zheng* (N-HN-20), *Xia Guan* (St 7), and *He Gu* (LI 4) were used. After acupuncture, direct moxibustion with wheat-sized cones or grains was performed mainly on *Zu San Li* (St 36), *Shen Shu* (Bl 23), *Yang Ling Quan* (GB 34), *Bi Guan* (St 31), *Shao Chong* (Ht 9), *Shao Ze* (SI 1), and the well points on the affected side of the upper and lower extremities. However, scarring was avoided. Three to five grains of moxa were administered at each point. Moxibustion was done once every other day, with 10 applications of moxa regarded as one course. Three days of rest were allowed between each successive course. Only standard acupuncture was performed at the above acupoints in members of the comparison group. No electrical stimulation or moxibustion was used on these patients.

The total effectiveness rates for the treatment and comparison group was 99.02% and 77.45% respectively (P< 0.005). According to the author of this study, contemporary medical experiments and clinical studies have shown that electro-acupuncture has several functions. First, by dilating the cranial blood vessels, it lowers the friction of the surrounding vessels. As a result, cranial blood flow is increased. Secondly, it lowers blood lipoproteins, enabling the body to absorb the accumulated fatty substances. Gradually this resolves thrombi and lowers blood viscosity. Third, the strong electrical stimulation experienced during the retention of the needles enhances local blood circulation. Muscular atrophy can be avoided and restoration of the nervous function can be enhanced. In short, electrical stimulation has the effect of quickening the blood and freeing the flow of the channels. As a result, qi and blood are regulated and rectified.

In the *Shen Jiu Jing Lun (Godly Moxibustion Classic Discussion),* it is said:

> Using the acrid property of *Ai Ye* (Folium Artemisiae Argyii) in moxibustion frees the flow of the 12 channels and enters the three yins. It regulates the qi and blood and cures the hundreds of diseases.

Therefore, direct moxibustion can regulate yin, yang, qi, and blood. It can also quicken the blood and transform stasis by disinhibiting the channels and opening the network vessels. In addition, *Zu San Li* fortifies the spleen and stomach and regulates the qi and blood. *Yang Ling Quan* strengthens the sinews and bones. The 12 well points free the flow of the network vessels. When these acupoints are stimulated with direct moxibustion, the restoration of bodily functions can be enhanced.

Cutaneous Needling with Scalp Acupuncture[58]

The following clinical trial, cutaneous needling and cupping are used in combination to reinforce the effectiveness of scalp acupuncture in treating apoplectic hemiplegia. Of 68 patients enrolled in this study, 45 were male and 23 were female. The youngest age was 23 years old and the oldest was 75 years of age. The shortest duration from the onset of stroke was one day and the longest was 90 days. Eighteen of these patients had hypertension, while 50 had normal blood pressure. In terms of type of stroke, eight patients had cerebral hemorrhage, 14 had cerebral infarction, and 46 had cerebral thrombosis. Thirty-one out of the 68 patients were examined by CT scan. Scalp acupuncture consisted of inserting 1.5 inch needles quickly at a 40 degree angle into the scalp. In order to increase the stimulation of an area, corresponding head areas were also stimulated by needling. For instance, if a motor area was chosen, then the upper, middle, and lower points were all administered. The needles were first applied at the lower point (*e.g.*, Facial Area), then at the middle point (*e.g.*, Upper Limb Area), and finally at the upper point (*e.g.*, Lower Limb and Trunk Area). The needles were all pointed upward, and all three needles were lined up in a straight line. Scalp acupuncture was performed bilaterally. The needles were applied first to the healthy side and then to the affected side of the body. For example, if there was paralysis on the right side of the body due to stroke occurring in the left brain, three needles were first applied on the healthy side or right Motor Area. These were inserted from the lower point to the upper point in a straight line. The needles were then manipulated until qi was obtained. The same procedure was later repeated on the left Motor Area or the affected side. The needles were manipulated at a speed of 100-200 times per minute, and manipulation was done once every 10 minutes. The level of stimulation level, frequency of manipulation, needle retention time, and manipulation speed all depended on the patient's physical condition, age, sex, blood pressure, severity of the stroke, the duration of the illness, and vacuity and repletion of the viscera and bowels. The exact treatment method was chosen according to TCM pattern discrimination. However, normally, the manipulation frequency was 2-3 times during each treatment, and needles were retained in the body from 30-120 minutes.

Cutaneous acupuncture consisted of tapping the channels and head stimulation areas with a cutaneous needle. The degree of stimulation of cutaneous acupuncture ranged from low to medium to high. Low stimulation was defined as the tapping causing local skin erythema but no bleeding. Medium stimulation meant that the tapping did cause slight local bleeding the size of the tip of the needle. High stimulation resulted in local bleeding the size of grains of wheat. The head stimulation areas were then fire-cupped except on areas with hair. Those patients who had hypertension were tapped heavily on the Upper Motor Area, Upper Sensory Area, Upper Foot Motor and Sensory Area, and *Tai Yang* (M-HN-9). This quickly lowered the blood pressure.

The following combined applications were used: The Motor Area was combined with *Hua Tuo Jia Ji* (M-BW-35) and governing vessel points were according to the patient's symptoms of paralysis. For example, for paralysis of the upper extremities, points at the level of C5 and C6 and T1 and T2 vertebrae were chosen. For paralysis of the lower extremities, points at the level of T11, T12 and L1-4 were chosen. The Sensory Area and corresponding governing vessel points were combined. The Upper Motor Area point, Motor and Sensory Area, and the Upper Sensory Area point were combined with *Tai Yang* (M-HN-9) and *Bai Hui* (Gv 20). The Motor Area was combined with

corresponding governing vessel points. The Sensory Area was combined with *Tai Yang* (M-HN-9). The Liver and Gallbladder Area was combined with *Bai Hui* (GV 20), etc.

Acupuncture was administered once per day, with 10 days equaling one course of treatment. A second course was administered after three days of rest. Using this protocol, it was judged effective in 10 cases (14.7%) and remarkably effective in 34 cases (50%), while 22 cases (32.4%) were judged cured. Only two cases (2.9%) got no effect. Therefore, the total effectiveness rate was 97.1%.

According to the authors of this study, the governing vessel ascends to the brain, is the sea of yang channels, and unites the yang qi. *Bai Hui*, a point on this vessel, acts as the meeting place of yang and, therefore, governs all yang. When this acupoint is needled, it enhances the circulation of qi and blood, frees the flow of qi among the channels, and stimulates motor functions. *Tai Yang* is among the first choices for brain diseases. It frees the flow of the channels and smoothes the circulation of qi and blood. Bleeding this point using cutaneous acupuncture quickly lowers blood pressure, arouses the spirit, and opens the orifices, calms the spirit and extinguishes liver wind. The paravertebral points regulate the viscera and bowels. They also treat diseases related to the viscera and bowels. Scalp acupuncture, the primary treatment method used in this study, was supplemented with cutaneous acupuncture and cupping which reinforced the effects of acupuncture by locally freeing the flow of the channels and allowing an abundance of qi and blood flow. Because cupping has the functions of quickening and moving blood, stopping pain, dispersing swelling and scattering binding or nodulations, it reinforces the effectiveness of scalp acupuncture in treating apoplectic hemiplegia.

Acupuncture Treatment for the Acute Stage of Stroke

The studies below both present research protocols for the treatment of the acute stage of stroke. In the first study, *Jing Ming* (Bl 1) was used to rapidly restore mobility to paralyzed limbs by bringing qi to the affected areas.[59] In many cases of acute stroke, the effects occurred within one minute. A total of 220 patients were randomly divided into two groups—a treatment and comparison group. The treatment group consisted of 120 patients 28-72 years of age. All these patients had suffered a stroke within the past three days. One hundred eight had cerebral thrombosis, while 12 had cerebral embolism. In the comparison group, there were 100 patients 30-78 years of age. Ninety-one of these patients had cerebral thrombosis and nine had cerebral embolism. There was no significant statistical difference between the treatment and comparison groups (P>0.05).

All patients from both groups were treated with standard Western medicine by neurologists. Western medical treatments included the administration of mannitol, ATP, and CoA intravenous drips once per day. Those patients with complications were treated accordingly. In addition, the treatment group received acupuncture on *Jing Ming* (Bl 1) using 0.35 millimeters in diameter and 50 millimeters long needles. *Jing Ming* was needled perpendicularly to a depth of 25 millimeters or until the bottom of the orbit was reached. No pulling, thrusting, or other manipulation of the needles was performed, and the needles were retained for one hour. One minute after the insertion, the subjects were asked to elevate their affected lower limb(s). Those capable of elevating their lower limb(s) to at least 60-90 degrees were asked to get up from their beds and walk around while still retaining the needle(s).

When the needle(s) was/were about to be taken out, three procedural steps were adopted. Step one: 1/3 of the needle was withdrawn and the surrounding area was pressed for one minute. Step two: step one was repeated, withdrawing the second 1/3 of the needle. Step three: the whole needle was removed and the area was pressed for three minutes to prevent bleeding. Treatment was done once per day, with 10 treatments equaling one course after which outcomes were analyzed.

In the comparison group, in addition to the standard Western medical treatments, patients were given Japanese-made DF-521 every other day. DF-521 is a strong thrombolytic. It is known as an effective medication showing fast results for stroke. On the first day, 10 units of DF-521 were added to 100ml of a 0.9% NS solution. The drip lasted an hour. On the third and fifth days, five units of DF-521 were added to this drip. The drip again lasted an hour. DF-521 was used three times in total. Outcomes were analyzed after 10 days.

The rate of reduction of cerebral edema was examined using CT scan. There was no significant difference in this rate between the treatment group (98.3%) and the comparison group (97.0%). There was also no significant difference in the evaluation of myodynamia of the lower limbs and functional recovery between the treatment group (90.0%) and the comparison group (91.0%). However, after the first series of treatments in the treatment group, 46 patients (38.3%) were able to walk independently compared to only 21 patients (21.0%) in the comparison group being able to do so. The table on the next page shows the differences in immediate efficacy between the two groups.

Further, in the treatment group, 18 were unconscious at the time of initial treatment

Group	#Patients	1 minute	2 minutes	1 hour	2 hours	No effect
Treatment	120	72	38	8	0	2
Comparison	100	0	0	12	83	5

and one patient died within 10 days. After treatment, the rest regained consciousness. In the comparison group, 16 patients were unconscious at the time of initial treatment and two cases died within 10 days. After treatment, 12 patients regained consciousness and two remained comatose.

According to Dr. Wang, the mechanism by which needling *Jing Ming* for one minute can bring an immediate response is still unclear. From the point of view of biomedicine, when cerebral thrombosis in a blood vessel reaches a certain stage, the affected tissues in the brain are deprived of oxygen and blood. As a result, the cerebral tissue caused the blood vessel spasm, leading to complete blockage. It is thought that needling *Jing Ming* lessens spasms of the blood vessels by regulating their circulation via the autonomic nerves. Hence, the auto-regulatory function of the blood circulation is restored and enhanced and blood can reach the blocked area. Therefore, the patients were able to walk after being needled.

From the point of view of TCM, all 12 regular channels in a human directly or indirectly flow to or connect with the eyes. When needles are deeply inserted at *Jing Ming* to near the bottom of the orbital socket, there is only a thin bone separating it from the brain. It is also the starting point of the bladder channel which circulates along the head to the back of the neck and thence to the back of the body. This channel also enters and connects with the brain. Two reasons have been posited why the patients were able to walk after needling

Jing Ming. First, it coincides with the principle that, "When a channel passes through a diseased area, [that channel] can treat [that area]." Second, the starting acupoint of a channel has a sufficiency of channel qi and an abundance of qi and blood. Therefore, deep insertion at *Jing Ming* is able to bring the needle qi to the affected area. It was noticed that the effectiveness diminished if the insertion was less than 25 millimeters in depth.

After needling *Jing Ming*, six patients sustained a hematoma in the local area. This may be due to puncturing of the small, superficial vessels close to the area. Normally, the swelling was absorbed after one day, leaving local bruises for about one week but not causing any damage to the eye. The deep blood vessels inside the eye have slippery surfaces; therefore, the needle normally slides past these. In terms of efficacy, DF-521 showed an effect an hour after administration. The condition of the subjects did not continue to improve after finishing the medication on the fifth day. On the other hand, deep insertion on *Jing Ming* started to show an effect after a minute. This effect increased daily during the series of treatments. In terms of cost, DF-521 was expensive while acupuncture was inexpensive. Therefore, deep insertion on *Jing Ming* is recommended for treating acute stages of stroke.

The second study in this section used fire needle technique.[60] Altogether, there were 128 cases of acute stroke enrolled in this two-wing comparison study. There were 66 cases of acute cerebral infarction which were treated using fire needle technique combined with medication and 62 cases of acute cerebral infarction treated using only medication. All the patients included in this study were scanned by cranial CT before treatment to exclude cases of cerebral hemorrhage. Also, those subjects with severe heart, liver, and kidney dysfunctions, in a coma, or already receiving treatment using anticlotting or thrombolytic medications were excluded from this study. Of the 66 patients in the treatment group, 38 were male and 28 were female. The average age was 62 years. The shortest duration since the onset of stroke was less than two hours and the longest was one week prior to the study. Twenty-four patients suffered from mild nerve damage, 33 from medium nerve damage, and nine from severe nerve damage. In the comparison group, there were 35 males and 27 females with an average age of 60 years. The shortest duration from the onset of stroke in this group was 12 hours and the longest was one week. There were 21 cases of mild nerve damage, 32 cases of medium nerve damage, and nine cases of severe nerve damage in this group. All patients in both groups were diagnosed by TCM practitioners based on symptoms and tongue examination. Patients either presented with qi vacuity and blood stasis or wind phlegm blocking the network vessels.

In the treatment group, *Bai Hui* (GV 20), *Chi Ze* (Lu 5), and *Wei Zhong* (Bl 40) were bled superficially once per day with 10 treatments equaling one course. A second course of treatment was begun after one day's rest. This treatment was supplemented with five units of plasmin (fibrinolysin) added to 250 milliliters of saline solution given as an intravenous drip. This medication was administered once per day for three days. In the comparison group,

patients were given 10 units of plasmin (fibrinolysin) added to 250 milliliters of saline solution. This intravenous drip was administered once per day for 20 days continuously. Depending on their condition, members of both the treatment and comparison groups were treated to lower cranial pressure to regulate blood pressure during this study period. Evaluations of all patients' nerve functions were done before and after treatment (on the 10th and 20th days). Proserozyme time (PT) and fibrinogen (FIB) were recorded before and after treatment (on the first, third, and tenth days). Blood, urine, liver, and kidney functions were tested for abnormalities.

The total effectiveness rate of 93.9% for the treatment group was higher than the 83.9% of the comparison group. This difference was statistically significant (P<0.05). In terms of TCM pattern discrimination in the treatment group, the total effectiveness for those presenting wind phlegm was higher (97.2%) than those presenting with qi vacuity and blood stasis (90.4%). The difference was not significant in the comparison group. The total effectiveness between the qi vacuity and blood stasis and the wind phlegm group was 83.3% and 84.4% respectively. The length of treatment needed in the treatment group was shorter than that in the comparison group. For example, it took 20 days in the treatment group to achieve basic cure; whereas, it took 27 days in the comparison group. The earlier treatment started after the stroke, the better the results. Also, the treatment group fared better than the comparison group in this regard. For example, the total effectiveness rates were 96.9% and 86.7% for the treatment and comparison groups respectively when treatment was started within three days. The total effectiveness in the two dropped to 87.0% and 78.3% respectively when treatment was started within seven days. The t- value of PT before and after the treatments was 1.83 for both groups. This difference was significant (P<0.05). The t-value of FIB was 1.726 for both groups and this difference was also significant (P<0.05).

According to the authors of this study, the disease mechanism of early stage stroke is blockage caused by blood stasis in the network vessels of the brain. Fire needle technique frees the flow of the channels and quickens the network vessels by warming the channels and scattering cold. In addition, bleeding the network vessels is a common treatment method in acupuncture. There are several reasons why *Bai Hui (GV 20)* was chosen. First, it belongs to the governing vessel which ascends to the brain. Second, the governing vessel is one of the eight extraordinary vessels. Third, *Bai Hui*, known as the sea of yang channels, is the meeting point of all three hand and foot yang channels where they ascend to the head. Additionally, the qi and blood enter and exit at both *Bai Hui* and *Feng Fu* (GV 16). The disease mechanism of blood stasis in the brain, the sea of marrow, usually takes place at *Bai Hui*. All these reasons explain why this point was chosen for the fire needling technique. *Chi Ze* (Lu 5) and *Wei Zhong* (Bl 40) were also bled to strengthen the functions of freeing the flow of the network vessels and quickening the blood. As stated above, the total effectiveness rate was higher in the wind phlegm group than in the qi vacuity and blood stasis group. This is because fire needle technique is a draining method and, therefore, is more effective in repletion patterns of stroke. The effectiveness of plasmin in the treatment of acute stroke has been confirmed. Using it in combination with fire needling technique strengthens its function, which lengthens the PT and lowers the FIB.

Endnotes

[1] Wu Yi-shin *et al.*, "The Treatment of 197 Cases of Cerebrovascular Disease Via Acupuncture at *Ren Ying* (St 9)," *Zhong Guo Zhen Jiu (Chinese Acupuncture & Moxibustion)*, #2, 1982, p. 9-10

[2] Warning: *Ren Ying* (St 9) is located at the bifurcation of the internal and external carotid arteries by the superficial anterior jugular vein, and medial to the internal jugular vein. Without understanding the regional anatomy or without using a careful, gentle technique, it is very easy to cause bleeding which is dangerous to the patient at this point. Beginners *must* be supervised when needling this point and should *not* attempt to needle this point just by reading this book.

[3] When applying pressure to stop bleeding, one should use light pressure and be gentle because the sympathetic trunk and vagus nerve lie at the deepest position of *Ren Ying*. Heavy pressure here can elicit a nerve reaction causing fainting or nausea.

[4] Wang Ke-jian *et al.*, "A Clinical Study on Using the *Yang Ming* Method to Treat Recovering Stroke Patients," *Zhong Guo Zhen Jiu (Chinese Acupuncture & Moxibustion)*, #1, 1996, p. 15-18

[5] Class 0: Able to return to work and manage housework

Class I: Able to live independently, able to partially return to work

Class II: Basically able to live independently, needing a small amount of help

Class III: Able to take care of oneself partially, but needs help from someone for most matters

Class IV: Able to work, but may need help at any time

Class V: Bed-ridden, able to sit in bed but needs help for all matters

Class VI: Bed-ridden with a certain degree of consciousness

Class VII: Comatose in a vegetative condition

[6] Twenty milliliters of blood was extracted from each patient before breakfast to measure their overall blood viscosity, the viscosity of

plasma and platelets, the formation of blood clots, and their lengths and weight (hydrated and dehydrated).

[7] Ultrasound equipment, TCZB -TCD, produced by a German company (EME) was used. Categories tested include ACA, MCA, PCA, T-ICA, SV, CURSOR, MV, PI, etc.

[8] Li Yu-ling *et al.*, "The Treatment of 162 Cases of Stroke Patients with Running Needles Along Yin Channels," *Shang Hai Zhen Jiu Za Zhi (Shanghai Journal of Acupuncture & Moxibustion)*, #6, 1994, p. 245

[9] In the original article this point is identified as *Zhong Ji (i.e.,* CV 3). We believe this is a typographical error since the use of running needle to connect these two points makes no sense. In our opinion, the correct point should read *Ji Quan* (Ht 1), and then one needle can connect the two points. Warning: Lateral to the point *Ji Quan* is the axillary artery. If the running needle goes to *Jian Yu* (LI 15), the insertion is very deep. Therefore, the practitioner must take special care to avoid piercing local blood vessels or nerves.

[10] *Ci Liao* (Bl 32) is located in the second posterior sacral foramen, along with the posterior branches of the second sacral nerves. Warning: Avoid damaging the nerve when using a deep insertion running needle technique here.

[11] *Shang Lian Quan* is an extra point located along the conception channel, one unit above the laryngeal prominence, in the depression between the margin of the mandible and the hyoid bone in the mylohyoid muscle, between geniohyoid muscle and the root of the tongue. Also located here are the lingual artery and vein, lingual nerve and a branch of the sublingual nerve. Warning: For such complex anatomy, deep insertion using a running needle should be done very carefully to avoid piercing the vessels and the nerves. If a hematoma appears, it can cause breathing difficulties and be a risk to the patient.

[12] The author of the original article does not mention which points in each pair were connected to the positive and negative leads.

[13] The four categories were 1) basically cured,

2) markedly effective, 3) improved, and 4) no effect. Basically cured meant that the muscular function of the four limbs reached or nearly reached stage V according to Brunnstrom's classification. Sensation returned to normal, speech was clear, and the patients were able to perform regular physical activities. Markedly effective meant that there was improvement in speech, the function of the four limbs reached stage III-IV, and the patients were able to take care of themselves. Improved meant that the extent of improvement of the function of the four limbs was more than one stage. The subjects, however, were not able to take care of themselves. No effect meant that there was no significant improvement in the muscular function of the four limbs after treatment.

[14] The total effectiveness rate = basically cured + markedly effective + improved.

[15] Cao Dai *et al.*, "A Clinical Study on the Leverage-interception Method in the Treatment of Ischemic Stroke," *Zhong Guo Zhen Jiu (Chinese Acupuncture & Moxibustion)*, #9, 2002, p. 591-593

[16] Ma Dan-yang was a great physician of the Jin dynasty. He was the author of Tian Xing Shi Er Xue Dan Chuo Fa *(The Song of the Twelve Heavenly Star Points for the Treatment of Disease)* which was first published in the 12th century *Yu Long Jing (Jade Dragon Classic)*. A twelfth point, *Tai Chong* (Liv 3) was added by Xu Feng in his work, the *Zhen Jiu Da Quan (Complete Collection of Acupuncture & Moxibustion)*.

[17] Chen Xiao-kai *et al.*, Clinical Observations on the Curative Effect of Needling Paravertebral Points on Hemiplegia after Cerebrovascular Accident," *Shang Hai Zhen Jiu Za Zhi (Shanghai Journal of Acupuncture & Moxibustion)*, #10, 2003, p. 9-10

[18] Cured meant that the hemiplegia had basically disappeared. Patients were able to walk and run and could live independently. Upper and lower muscular strength was restored to IV or above. Marked effect was defined as marked improvement in the symptoms of hemiplegia. The patients were able to walk and upper and lower muscular strength

improved two levels or more. Some effect meant that the symptoms of hemiplegia had improved somewhat, while muscular strength had improved one level or more. No effect meant that there was no obvious improvement in the hemiplegia or associated symptoms after treatment.

[19] Total effectiveness rate = cured + marked effect + some effect

[20] Yuan Jin-long, "Indicators of Changes in Stroke Patient's Tongue Appearance for Differential Classification," *Gan Su Zhong Yi (Gansu Chinese Medicine)*, #5, 2001, p. 1-2

[21] Two separate classifications, protruding tongue and rigid tongue, were combined from the original article due to their similarity.

[22] Guan Zun-hui, "Tongue Acupuncture (Part I)," *International Journal of Clinical Acupuncture*, #1, 2000, p. 31-35

[23] Guan Zun-hui, "Tongue Acupuncture (Part II)," *International Journal of Clinical Acupuncture*, #2, 2000, p. 125-128

[24] Li Jian-shan, "Tongue Acupuncture with Body Needles for Treatment Compared to Only Using Body Acupuncture," *Lin Chuang Zhen Jiu Za Zhi (Journal of Clinical Acupuncture & Moxibustion)*, #5, 1995, p. 33-34

[25] Chen Sin-seng, "The Treatment of 120 Hemiplegia Stroke Cases with Awn Needle Acupuncture Along With a Comparison Group," *Lin Chuang Zhen Jiu Za Zhi (Journal of Clinical Acupuncture & Moxibustion)*, #6, 1995, p. 4-5

[26] This acupoint is created for use with awn needle acupuncture. Its location is two inches inferior to the mastoid process, posterior to the border of muscle sternocleidomastoid (SCM) and one inch anterior and inferior to *Tian You* (TB 16).

[27] Warning: The anatomy of the neck is complicated and acupuncture on the neck has high risk, especially if using deep insertion. Practitioners should not attempt this technique by just reading this article. They learn how to needle this point from someone who has experience with it. The purpose of this article is to simply introduce the knowledge of a special technique to treat hemiplegia.

[28] Lu Shou-kang *et al.*, "A Special Needling Technique," *One Hundred Techniques of Acupuncture*, China Medical Science, Beijing, First Edition Oct. 1987, p. 146. This technique is one of five techniques traditionally indicated for treating painful muscles. It consists of first needling perpendicularly and then obliquely to one side and the other.

[29] Zhou Li-li *et al.*, "Awn Needle Acupuncture in the Treatment of 27 Cases of the Sequelae of Stroke," *Shang Hai Zhen Jiu Za Zhi (Shanghai Journal of Acupuncture & Moxibustion)*, #4, 1991, p. 12

[30] Sun Mao-bin, "Discussion of Using Wrist-Ankle Needling Technique to Treat Hemiplegia Stroke Patients," *World United Journal For Traditional Chinese Medicine and Acupuncture*, June, 1998, p. 3

[31] Upper One is located on the ulnar side of the ulna. It is in the depression between the ulnar bone and the tendon of the muscle flexor carpi ulnaris.

[32] Upper Five is located in the space between the radius and the ulna on the dorsal side of the wrist.

[33] Lower One is located in the medial aspect of the tendon calcaneus.

[34] Lower Six is located on the lateral border of the tendons of the muscle calcaneus.

[35] Insert another needle from the tip of the first needle at Upper Five or Lower One. The second needle should follow the vertical axes of the limbs moving in the same direction as the first needle.

[36] Lian Han-jian *et al.*, "Clinical Observations on the Treatment of Apoplectic Hemiplegia by Magnetic-field Electric Pulse Point Stimulation," *Shang Hai Zhen Jiu Za Zhi (Shanghai Journal of Acupuncture & Moxibustion)*, #4, 2000, p. 18-19

[37] Brunnstrom's classification is based on the mobility function of upper and lower extremities. It is graded with six stages (I, II, III, IV, V and VI). The higher stage indicates better mobility of the extremities. However the extent of improvement is measured by the extent of changes through the various stages. For example, improvement is regarded as good from stage III or below to stage V or above.

[38] Zhang Xiao-li, "Magnetic Acupoint Therapy in the Treatment of 116 Cases of the Sequelae of Cerebral Thrombosis," *Zhong Guo Zhen Jiu (Chinese Acupuncture & Moxibustion)*, #4, 1997, p. 227-228

[39] Wah Yan-ling *et al.*, "The Clinical Application of Crowded Needling Technique," *Shang Hai Zhen Jiu Za Zhi (Shanghai Journal of Acupuncture & Moxibustion)*, #6, 1982, p. 22-24

[40] There are six acupoints on the left and six on the right of *Feng Fu* (GV 16). Adding *Feng Fu, Ya Men* (GV 15), and *Nao Hu* (GV 17), there are 15 points altogether.

[41] Warning: The anatomy of the neck is complicated. These acupoints are close to both the medulla oblongata or brainstem and the spinal cord. Therefore, deep insertion at these locations carries high risk. In addition, the practitioner must take extreme care with the direction of needle insertion. It should not be upward into the medulla oblongata where it could cause death, since the medulla is the area that regulates the heart and respiration.

[42] Warning: After needle insertion, it is best if the patient feels localized distention. If the patient feels a strong electric sensation, it could mean that the spinal cord has been touched and the needle should be removed immediately.

[43] Wang Jin *et al.*, "Using the Setting the Mountain on Fire Technique to Treat 49 Cases of Bodily Dysfunction Due to Stroke," *Shang Hai Zhen Jiu Za Zhi (Shanghai Journal of Acupuncture & Moxibustion)*, #2, 1994, p. 63

[44] This formula consists of: *Huang Qi* (Radix Astragali), *Dang Gui* (Radix Angelicae Sinensis), *Chuan Xiong* (Rhizoma Chuanxiong), *Chi Shao* (Radix Paeoniae Rubrae), *Tao Ren* (Semen Persicae), *Hong Hua* (Flos Carthami), and *Di Long* (Pheretima)

[45] Lai Feng-shan *et al.*, "A Clinical Study on Acupuncture Based on Timing in the Treatment of Ischemic Stroke," *Zhong Guo Zhen Jiu (Chinese Acupuncture & Moxibustion)*, #1, 1992, p. 1-4

[46] Hu Jian-bei *et al.*, *The Quick Reference Flying & Soaring Eight Methods Time Table,*

Anhui Science & Technology Press, Hefei, 1990, p. 32

[47] Qiu Mou-liang, *Zhen Jiu Xue (The Study of Acupuncture & Moxibustion)*, Shanghai Science & Technology Press, Shanghai, 1985, p. 212-213

[48] Of the 63 patients in this study, 90.63% had various degrees of nail fold microcirculation problems. These included increased permeability of the micrangium, distortion of the microscopic blood vessels, slowing of blood circulation, and irregular, shortened blood vessels.

[49] This includes platelet stickiness and concentration, blood clot formation, clot retraction time, overall blood stickiness, etc.

[50] Zhang Deng-bu, "The Moxibustion Treatment of CHD and CVA," *International Journal of Clinical Acupuncture,* #3, 1996, p. 285-287

[51] Li Zhi-xiang *et al.*, "The Treatment of 210 Cases of Post Cerebrovascular Disease by First Needling the Healthy Side and Then the Affected Side," *International Journal of Clinical Acupuncture*, #1, 1993, p. 33-34

[52] Zhou Bao-min, "The Treatment of 228 Cases of the Sequelae of Stroke by Placing Herbal Patches on Acupoints," *Shang Hai Zhen Jiu Za Zhi (Shanghai Journal of Acupuncture & Moxibustion)*, #2, 1991, p. 15

[53] Tan Wen-lan, "A Clinical Study of the Acupoint Hot Rubbing Method on 207 Cases of Apoplectic Hemiplegia Due To Cerebral Infarction," *Gan Su Zhong Yi (Gansu Chinese Medicine)*, #9, 2003, p. 30-31

[54] Liu Xie-hua, "Using *He Gu* Needling on *Shou San Li* (LI 10) & *Fu Tu* (St 32) for the Treatment of Stroke," *Zhong Guo Zhen Jiu (Chinese Acupuncture & Moxibustion)*, #8, 1997, p. 479-480

[55] The six levels of muscular strength used to grade outcomes in this study included:

Level 0: There was no contraction of the muscles.

Level 1: There was slight contraction in the muscles but no mobility of the joints.

Level 2: The muscles were able to contract to move the joints but they could not resist pulling.

Level 3: The muscles contracted only in resistance to pulling.

Level 4: The muscles were able to contract from both resistance against pulling as well as slight resistance.

Level 5: The muscles were able to resist strong resistance. In other words, the muscular strength was judged normal.

[56] Muscular strength in the affected limbs was compared before and after treatment. When the muscular strength increased by one level, the treatment was regarded as effective. When the muscular strength increased to two or more levels, the treatment was regarded as remarkably effective.

[57] Zeng Jie-hong, "Observations on the Effectiveness of Electro-acupuncture with Wheat Grains of Moxibustion for Treating the Sequelae of Stroke," *Shang Hai Zhen Jiu Za Zhi (Shanghai Journal of Acupuncture &*

Moxibustion), #1, 2000, p. 22

[58] Jin Jie *et al.*, "Clinical Observations on Combining Cutaneous Acupuncture with Scalp Acupuncture in the Treatment of 68 Cases of Apoplectic Hemiplegia," *Proceedings of The First International Conference on the Chinese Micro-acupuncture Therapy*, San Francisco, 1995, p. 40-41

[59] Wang Shou-ping, "Observations on Deep Insertion at *Jing Ming* (Bl 1) to Treat Acute Stroke," *Zhong Guo Zhen Jiu (Chinese Acupuncture & Moxibustion)*, #7, 2000, p. 405-406

[60] Zhang Jie *et al.*, "Recent Observations on the Effectiveness of Fire Needle Technique as the Main Method for the Treatment of Acute Cerebral Infarction," *Zhong Guo Zhen Jiu (Chinese Acupuncture & Moxibustion)*, #3, 2000, p. 151-152

SIX
Acupuncture Treatments for Various Specific Post-stroke Symptoms

In clinical practice, stroke patients usually present a complicated set of symptoms. Acupuncture ideally helps patients as a whole, but there are some symptoms which are more difficult to treat. These post-stroke symptoms typically linger even after the relief of other symptoms. This chapter introduces a survey of 23 unique treatment methods for such persistent post-stroke symptoms. Clinical studies show faster recovery with these special treatments.

1. Depression

Depression is a commonly seen condition in post-stroke patients. Its symptoms include bad mood, emotional lability, low self-esteem, loss of appetite, and loss of interest for the things the patient had previously enjoyed or been enthusiastic about. Its most common subjective symptoms are hopelessness, helplessness, and loss of self-esteem, and these factors severely influence the patient's quality of life and his or her recovery from stroke. Therefore, practitioners should not misdiagnose nor forget to treat this condition. In the following clinical trial, 60 post-stroke patients with depression were treated in a hospital out-patient clinic and during home visits.[1] Within this group, there were 42 males and 18 females aged 52-70 years. In 32 of these cases, stroke was caused by infarction on the left side of the brain, and in eight cases, it was caused by infarction on the right side. In 13 cases, stroke was caused by left brain hemorrhage, and in the other seven cases, it was caused by right brain hemorrhage. All patients were diagnosed as depressed according to the criteria for unipolar depression in the *IDC-10 (International Disease Classification, 10th edition)*. Stroke had been diagnosed by clinical symptoms and brain CT scan. The symptoms of depression had arisen only after the occurrence of stroke and the symptoms of depression improved with recovery from CVA. There was no evidence for the cause of depression from any other reason besides stroke. The severity of depression was gauged by the Hamilton Depression Scale (HAMD Scale). This required a score of 20 points or more before patients were chosen for inclusion in this clinical trial. The 60 patients enrolled in this study were randomly divided into two groups—a treatment group and a comparison group.

All members of the treatment group received electro-acupuncture on only two points: *Bai Hui* (GV 20) and *Yin Tang* (M-HN-3). At *Bai Hui,* the tip of the needle was inserted anteriorly and obliquely to approximately 7-10 millimeters in depth. At *Yin Tang*, the insertion was directed superior to the same depth as *Bai Hui*. The two needles were connected to a G6805 electro-acupuncture device using six volt intermittent waves and a frequency of two Hertz. Intensity was adjusted to the patient's tolerance, with the soft tissue slightly pulsing to the intermittent wave. Treatment was given once per day for 40 minutes, with six weeks equaling one course of therapy. All members of the comparison group were treated with standard acupuncture technique at *Bai Hui* (GV 20), *Yin Tang* (M-HN-3), *Nei Guan* (Per 6) and *Shen Men* (Ht 7). Supplementation hand technique was used at each point for approximately one minute, after which the needles were retained for 40 minutes. Treatment was given once per day, with six weeks also equaling one course.

The analysis of study outcomes were made by a doctor who did not perform the acupuncture treatments. This doctor used HAMD, Zung Self-rating Depression Scale (SDS), and Clinical Assessment Geriatric Scale (SCAG) to check patients before and after treatment. Based on changes in HAMD scores, eight of the treatment group showed a marked effect, 19 got some effect, and three cases got no effect for a total effectiveness rate of 90%. In the comparison group, 17 cases got some effect and 13 cases got no effect. None showed a marked effect. The effectiveness rate in this group was only 56.7%. SDS analysis and SCAG analysis both also showed significant differences in effectiveness rates between the treatment and comparison groups.

Therefore, the authors of this study were satisfied with this electro-acupuncture technique to treat the patients with post-stroke depression. Further, it is simple to apply and produced no side effects.

In the next study, there were 60 post-stroke patients diagnosed by CT scan or MRI.[2] Thirty of these patients were randomly assigned to the treatment group and the other 30 patients were in the comparison group. In the treatment group, there were 19 males and 11 females with an average age of 61.5 years. Nine of these cases of stroke were caused by hemorrhage and 21 were caused by infarction. The time since the onset of stroke in this group averaged 1.8 years. The duration of depression averaged 1.1 years. In the comparison group, there were 16 males and 14 females with an age average of 58.9 years. Stroke was caused by hemorrhage in six of these cases and by infarction in 24 cases. The time since onset of stroke in this group averaged 1.9 years, and the duration of depression averaged one year. Based on this data, these two groups were judged suitable for comparison in this clinical trial. All these stroke patients showed the typical symptoms of depression and their HAMD score was above 20 points each. Criteria for exclusion from this study included failing the HAMD test due to side effects from some of the antihypertension drugs or confusion in the patient.

All members of the treatment group received acupuncture at the main points *Bai Hui* (GV 20), *Shang Xing* (GV 23), *Yin Tang* (M-HN-3), *Ren Zhong* (GV 26), *Shang Zhong* (CV 17), and *Jiu Wei* (CV 15). Auxiliary points included *Feng Long* (St 40), *Zhong Wan* (CV 12), *Tai Xi* (Ki 3), *Qi Men* (Liv 14), and *Yang Ling Quan* (GB 34). After the qi was obtained, supplementation, drainage, or even supplementing-even draining hand technique was applied based on each patient's pattern discrimination. The needles were retained for 30 minutes, and treatment was done once per day, with six treatments per week. After one day of rest, treatments were resumed and continued for another four weeks. All members of the comparison group were administered 20 milligrams of Prozac® 1-2 times per day for four weeks. Both groups received the same standard Western medical treatment for the original symptoms of stroke.

Cure was defined as disappearance of the three main symptoms of depression, *i.e.*, emotional deterioration, bradyphrenia, and decrease of speech and movement. The patient was also very cooperative with the acupuncture treatment. Marked effect was defined as basic disappearance of the three main symptoms but interest in acupuncture treatment was low. Some effect was defined as improvement in symptoms but the patient was unable to actively participate in treatments to help daily life activities. No effect was defined as no change in symptoms. Based on these criteria, three cases in the treatment group were judged cured, 14 got a marked effect, nine cases got some effect, and four got no effect for a total effectiveness rate of 86.7% In the comparison group, two cases were judged cured, 12 got a marked effect, 10 got some effect, and six got no effect for a total effectiveness rate of 80.0%. Therefore, there was no significant statistical difference between the two groups in the total effectiveness rates (P> 0.05). However, in the treatment group, in five cases treatment took less than three days to show effect, in 12 cases it took 4-7 days, in seven cases it took 8-14 days, and in two cases it took 15-21 days. Thus the average time from the beginning of treatment to the appearance of effect in this group was eight days. In the comparison group, in four cases treatment took 4-7 days

to manifest some effect, in nine cases it took 8-14 days, in 10 cases it took 15-21 days, and in one case it took 22-28 days. The average time from the initiation of treatment to the manifestation of some effect in this group was 14.5 days. Hence there was a significant difference in the time taken to show therapeutic effect between the two groups (P< 0.05). Based on these outcomes, the author concluded that acupuncture has a good therapeutic effect with efficacy similar to Prozac®, but that it produces results faster and without side effects.

2. Dysfunction of the Thumb

Loss of function of the thumb caused by firm compression by the other four fingers is the most common post-stroke motor impairment of the upper extremities. After more than 10 years of working with stroke patients, Drs. Xie Tu-dun and Chou Bing from the Shanxi Medical University Second Affiliated Hospital have found an especially effective extra-channel point for the treatment of this condition. They named this point "Extending Thumb Point" and used it to treat 36 cases of this condition from 1999-2002.[3] Among these 36 patients there were 22 males and 14 females aged 41-76 years. The shortest time from the onset of stroke to the initiation of treatment was eight days, while the longest was one and a half years. Stroke was caused by hemorrhage in 11 cases and by ischemia in 25 cases. With the patient's elbow bent 90 degrees, a line was drawn from the tip of the elbow to the point *Yang Xi* (LI 5). Extending Thumb Point was located at the midpoint of this line. A needle was inserted perpendicularly to a depth of 0.3-0.5 inches. Then the needle was stimulated electrically with a discontinuous wave at a frequency of 120-180 times per minute. The intensity was to the level of the patient's tolerance, and the electrical impulse caused the thumb to move into the extended position. The needles were retained for 30-60 minutes per treatment, and the patient was treated daily, with 10 treatments equaling one course. Treatment was then stopped for one week of rest before starting the next course.

Marked effect meant that the motion of the thumb returned to normal and that the hand could carry and hold things naturally. Some effect meant that the motion of the thumb was fine, but its strength for moving and extending was still weak. No effect meant that the motion of the thumb was still restricted and there was no change in symptoms. Based on these criteria, 23 cases (63.9%) got a marked effect, 10 cases (27%) got some effect, and three cases (8.3%) got no effect.

The authors of this study based the discovery of this new extra-channel point on the musculature of the arm. The electrical stimulation creates an impulse to the paralyzed muscle fibers. These involuntary movements help the recovery of the motion and function of the thumb followed by recovery of the hand. From the authors' clinical observations, effective results were closely related to the duration of the stroke. In other words, as in so many other of the studies included in this book, the shorter the duration the better and the faster the results.

3. Dysfunction of the Wrist and Ankle Joints

Another common post-stroke complication is impaired joint function, and, among the joints that may be affected, recovery of the wrist and ankle joints is often troublesome. Based on the hypothesis that such impairment is due to blockage of the channels resulting in damage of the sinews, Ma

Guang-hao and his associates from Naval General Hospital in Beijing treated this complication with running needle technique on selected acupoints to relieve this blockage. In the following study, there were 46 patients who had impaired function of the wrist or ankle joints during the recovering phase of their strokes.[4] These patients were randomly divided into two groups—a treatment group and a comparison group. There were 26 patients in the treatment group and 20 in the comparison group. Fourteen of the patients in the treatment group were male, while 12 were female. In the comparison group, there were 12 males and eight females. The age range in both groups was 44-78 years. Similarly, the duration of stroke to the time of treatment was two weeks to three years in both groups. In terms of TCM pattern discrimination, nine patients in the treatment group presented with wind phlegm obstructing the network vessels, and there were seven patients in the comparison group who manifest the same pattern. The number of patients in each group who manifest ascendant liver yang hyperactivity were five and four respectively. Those who manifest phlegm heat bowel repletion were four and two respectively, those who presented with qi vacuity and blood stasis in both groups were six and five respectively, and those who presented with yin vacuity and stirring of wind in both groups were two and two. Therefore, there were no significant statistical difference in terms of sex, age, disease duration, or pattern discrimination between these two groups (P>0.05).

Range of motion (ROM) of the wrist was expressed as the average measurement of backwards flexion, palmar flexion, and radial and ulnar flexions, while ROM of the ankle was expressed as the average measurement of the backwards and metatarsal flexion of the ankle. Both the healthy and affected sides were measured for comparison. Impairment of the joint was classified according to its severity. Severe impairment meant that the ROM of the affected joint was less than 10% of the corresponding joint on the healthy limb. Moderate impairment meant that the ROM of the affected joint was 10-30% of the corresponding joint on the healthy limb. Mild impairment meant that the ROM of the affected joint was 30-60% of the corresponding joint on the healthy limb, and recovered meant that the ROM of the affected joint was more than 60% of the corresponding joint of the healthy limb. Patients whose ROM of the wrist or ankle joints of the affected limb were greater than 60% of that of the healthy limb were excluded from the study.

Patients in the treatment group received running needling by penetrating paired acupoints. The needles were inserted either vertically or horizontally up to two inches on four sets of acupoints as follows.

Wrist:

Yang Xi (LI 5)————→ *Yang Chi* (TB 4) horizontally
Wai Shen Men[5]————→*Da Ling* (Per 7) horizontally
Yang Chi (TB 4) ————→*Da Ling* (Per 7) vertically

Ankle:

Qiu Xu (GB 40)————→*Zhao Hai* (Ki 6)

Additional points were selected for given patients according to TCM pattern discrimination. For wind phlegm obstructing the network vessel, *Feng Chi* (GB 20), *Yin Ling Quan* (Sp 9), and *Feng Long* (St 40) were added. For ascendant liver yang hyperactivity, *Tai Chong* (Liv 3), *Tai Xi* (Ki 3), and *Yang*

Ling Quan (GB 34) were added. For phlegm heat bowel repletion, *Tian Shu* (St 25), *Feng Long* (St 40), and *Shang Ju Xu* (St 37) were added. For qi vacuity and blood stasis, *Qi Hai* (CV 6), *Zu San Li* (St 36), and *Xue Hai* (Sp 10) were added. For yin vacuity with stirring of wind, *Tai Chong* (Liv 3), *Tai Xi* (Ki 3), *Shen Shu* (Bl 23), and *Gan Shu* (Bl 18) were added. A 30 gauge 1.5-2 inch filiform needle was inserted into the first acupoint reaching towards the paired second acupoint until the tip of the needle could be felt under the skin. After the arrival of the qi, the needle was manipulated using even supplementing-even draining hand technique for one minute. For the additional acupoints based on TCM pattern discrimination, after the arrival of qi, the needle was manipulated with draining technique for the first three patterns and with supplementing technique for the last two patterns.

In the comparison group, the first point of each of the above pairs was used. Needles were inserted perpendicularly 0.5 inches at each point followed by manipulating as described above. Acupuncture needles were twisted once every 10 minutes in both groups and the needles were retained for 30 minutes each treatment. Treatment was given once per day, five days per week for six weeks.

In order to compare the treatment outcomes between the two groups, the authors devised a numeric system corresponding to the degree of ROM impairment. Severe impairment equaled three points, moderate impairment equaled two points, mild impairment equaled one point, and recovered equaled zero points. The therapeutic effect was expressed as the difference in ROM before and after treatment. Excellent effect equaled three points, good effect equaled two points, fair effect equaled one point, and no effect equaled zero points.

Based on these criteria, while no patients achieved complete recovery, *i.e.*, excellent effect, there were more patients in the treatment group with good and fair results than in the comparison group (P<0.05). In the treatment group, the total effectiveness rates were 73.1% for both back flexion and palm flexion, 53.8% for radial flexion, and 61.5% for ulnar flexion of the wrist joints. They were 65.4% for back flexion and 61.5% for metatarsal flexion of the ankle joints. The recovery of ROM of the wrist and ankle joints in the study group was far better than that of the comparison group (P<0.05). From the above outcomes, the authors concluded that the running needle technique generated sufficient qi to free the flow of the channels and provided nourishment to overcome the blockage which enabled the recovery of the lost function of the wrist and ankle joints.

4. Dysfunction of the Upper Extremity

One of the major sequelae of stroke is paralysis or partial paralysis of the upper extremity due to the lack of qi. This is caused by the stroke creating secondary qi stagnation and blood stasis in the channels in the affected extremity. In his study on post-stroke upper extremity dysfunction, Liu Zhen-chun used a T-shaped needling method to free the flow of the channels near the joints resulting in the restoration of flexibility and function.[6] The study included 42 patients, 29 males and 13 females, 2.5-83 years of age. These patients' course of disease ranged from 21 days to eight years. Twenty-seven patients in the study had a course of disease of 21 days to six months, 11 patients had suffered from six months to one year, and four patients had been affected 1-8 years.

The main and auxiliary points used in this study consisted of:

Jian Yu (LI 15) coupled with auxiliary point
Jian Zhen (SI 19)
Qu Chi (LI 11) coupled with
Chi Ze (Lu 5)
Yang Chi (TB 4) coupled with
Yang Xi (LI 5)
He Gu (LI 4) coupled with
Yu Ji (Lu 10)
Zhong Zhu (TB 32) coupled with auxiliary point
Hou Xi (SI 3)

With the patient sitting upright, the affected arm was bent and placed in front of his or her abdomen. The five main needles were inserted straight into *Jian Yu, Qu Chi, Yang Chi, He Gu,* and *Zhong Zhu,* and the qi was obtained. Then each of the auxiliary points was needled so that the body of each needle was at a 90 degree angle to its paired main point. Again the qi was obtained. Without further manipulation, the needles were retained for 30 minutes. Patients received one treatment per day with 10 days equaling one course. After three days of rest, a follow-up course of treatments commenced. In the study, patients received from 17-60 treatments.

If the muscle dynamics were restored to normal and every joint extended and bent freely, this was defined as cured. Marked effect meant that every joint extended and bent freely but the patient had difficulty with some tasks. Myodynamia had been raised more than two grades. Improved meant that myodynamia was somewhat raised, but the affected joints were still weak or slightly rigid. No effect meant that there was no apparent change after treatment. Based on these criteria, 17 patients were judged cured, 21 patients got a marked effect, one patient improved, and three patients got no effect. Therefore, the cure rate was 40.5% and the total effectiveness rate was 92.9%.

According to Dr. Liu, following stroke, the limbs become stiff due to blood vacuity failing to nourish them. Qi vacuity due to stroke also creates qi stagnation and blood stasis blocking the channels and network vessels throughout the limbs. The use of T-shaped needling on the shoulder, arm, and wrist helps to free the flow of the channels near these joints, thus allowing the qi and blood to circulate freely, nourish the area, and restore function to the limb.

5. Dysopsia

Post-stroke dysopsia is a disease of the cerebral blood vessels. It is a major complication in diseases of the occipital lobe of the cerebrum. Its clinical manifestations are hemianopia and decrease or loss of visual acuity. In recent years, Zhang Yu-lian and his associates from Tianjing College of Chinese Medicine Second Affiliated Hospital have adopted scalp acupuncture and periocular needling for the treatment of post-stroke dysopsia. In the following study, there were 36 patients.[7] Twenty-two of these were hospitalized and 14 were outpatients. Patients with eye diseases had been excluded through eye examination. All patients in this study had CT scans by which it was determined there were 16 cases of occipital lobe infarction, eight cases of parietal-occipital lobe infarction, four cases of temporal-occipital lobe infarction, six cases of temporal-parietal-occipital lobe infarction, and two cases of occipital lobe hemorrhage. Thirty-two of these patients were male and four were female. Their ages ranged from 46-72 years old. There were 21 cases with a course of disease under two weeks, nine cases with a course of disease between two weeks and one month, four cases with a course of disease between 1-2 months, and two cases with a course of disease more than two months. Further, there were 32 cases of hemianopsia, 28 cases of decreased visual acuity, and two cases of lost visual acuity.

In terms of scalp acupuncture, three needles were inserted 3-4 centimeters deep superior to the occiput. The middle point was centered above the occipital tuberosity and the other two points were one centimeter bilateral to this center point. The angle of insertion for scalp needles was at 15 degrees. Using rapid penetrating technique, the needles were inserted to the cutaneous level, then downward under the galea aponeurotica to a depth of 1.5-1.8 inches. According to the patient's condition, either the nine-six supplementation method, or drainage by lifting and thrusting method was applied up and down about one inch distance, followed by rapidly twisting the needles 180 degrees at a frequency of 200 times per minute for about 30 seconds.

Periocular acupuncture consisted of needling *Tai Yang* (M-HN-9), *Yang Bai* (GB 14), *Si Bai* (St 2), and *Jing Ming* (Bl 1). *Tai Yang* was needled 1.2 inches deep obliquely upward towards the back of the eye at about 15 degrees. *Yang Bai* was needled with a running needle to *Yu Yao* (M-HN-6). *Si Bai* and *Jing Ming* were needled perpendicularly. When inserting the needle at *Jing Ming*, the index finger of the left hand was used to push and stabilize the eye ball laterally. The depth was 1.2 inches, and no manipulation was performed. After the needle was withdrawn, pressure was applied with a small piece of cotton for more than one minute to prevent bleeding.

Treatment was done once per day, and one course consisted of five treatments. A total of four courses were administered with a two-day break between each successive course.

Cure was defined as a return to normal of both visual acuity and visual field. Marked

Duration	No.	Cured	Marked Effect	Some Effect	No Effect	Total Effect
<2 weeks	21	9	11	1	0	100%
2wks-1mo	9	2	5	2	0	100%
1mo-2mo	4	0	2	2	0	100%
>2months	2	0	0	1	1	50.00%
Total	36	11	18	6	1	97.2%

Table 1. Correlation between Duration of Disease and Efficacy

effect was defined as improvement in visual acuity by three grades or more with marked improvement in visual field which was still not at normal standards. Some effect was defined as improvement in visual acuity less than three grades and only some improvement in visual field. No effect meant that there was no noticeable change in visual acuity or visual field from before to after treatment. The table above shows the correlation between the duration of disease and treatment effects.

This table shows there is a close inverse relationship between the duration of disease and treatment efficacy. The next table shows mean changes in visual acuity before and after treatment.

Results also showed that, after needling, the ingress time was shortened, the egress time was lengthened, the alpha/beta value was reduced, and the amplitude was raised. Such results indicate that needling can increase blood circulation in the brain,

improve the intra-cranium blood supply, increase ingress/egress rating and lower the angio-resistance index. This, in turn, means that the elasticity of cerebral blood vessels is improved and external resistance is lowered, thus benefitting cerebral blood circulation. Further, it was clearly observed that, after needling, the amplitude of the intraorbital rheogram was raised, the rise time was shortened, the egress time was lengthened, the perfusion of blood flow index and the output index were increased, and the angio-resistance index was lowered. Hence it was concluded that scalp acupuncture plus peri-ocular acupoints can improve intraorbital blood supply of post-stroke dysopsia patients as well as the elasticity of intraorbital blood vessels.

According to the authors of the above study, the main cause of post-stroke dysopsia is infarction of blood vessels in the brain. Occasionally it is also caused by hemorrhage in the brain. The location of the disease is mainly in the cerebral occipital

Affected Eye	Number of Eyes	Visual Acuity Before Treatment	Visual Acuity After Treatment	P
Right	26	4.15±0.20	4.96±0.22	<0.01
Left	28	4.51±0.21	4.95±0.23	<0.01

Table 2. Change of Visual Acuity Before and After Needling

Time	Ingress Time(s)	Egress Time(s)	Alpha/Beta	Amplitude (Omega)
Before	0.113±0.008	0.699±0.035	0.173±0.007	0.126±0.007
After	0.094±0.007	0.800±0.025	0.120±0.013	0.150±0.009

Time	Ratio	Angio-resistance Index
Before	0.959±0.012	0.751±0.022
After	0.988±0.005	0.735±0.021

Table 3. Effects of Scalp Acupuncture Plus Periocular Acupoints on Patients' Rheoencephalogram (n=16)(x-bar ± s)

lobe. For this reason, regular body acupuncture with routine manipulation technique is usually not adequate. The acupuncture site for the three needles on the superior occipital is located at the visual center of the cerebral cortex. Needling at these three points can improve blood flow to the visual center at the occipital lobes. Thus it can improve the function of the visual cortex. Rheoencephalogram and intraorbital rheogram reflect to a certain degree, the condition of the blood supply of the cerebrum. Observation of the results of this study clearly indicate that needling the three superior occipital and the periocular acupoints can improve blood supply to the cerebrum and the intraorbital region of the eye. Hence, improvement in visual acuity and the visual field can be achieved. These results not only demonstrate the theory behind the treatment of post-stroke dysopsia with scalp acupuncture plus periocular acupuncture, they also provide the physiological basis for the clinical efficacy of such treatment.

6. Dysphagia

Difficulty swallowing impairment is another common symptom of stroke. According to statistics, this symptom exists in 20.9-64% of cases in the acute stage and in 6-29% of cases more than one month past onset. Difficulty swallowing affects the patient's absorption of nutrients and can also lead to inhalation pneumonia and suf-

Time	Ingress Time(s)	Egress Time(s)	Amplitude (Omega)
Before	0.094±0.009	0.640±0.072	0.076±0.010
After	0.090±0.010	0.660±0.069	0.084±0.012

Time	Perfusion Index	Output Index	Angio-resistance Index
Before	0.817±0.141	0.120±0.016	0.684±0.121
After	0.946±0.186	0.128±0.019	0.652±0.112

Table 4. Effects of Scalp Acupuncture Plus Periocular Acupoints on the Intraorbital Rheogram of Patients with Post-stroke Dysopsia

focation. In the first study presented below, Dr. Zong Tao and associates treated 88 cases of post-stroke difficulty swallowing.[8] The total number of cases enrolled in this two-wing comparison study was 128, all of whom were hospitalized stroke patients. All 128 patients met the diagnostic criteria of the national standard for the diagnosis of stroke in China. All patients had clear cognition and their vital signs were stable. These 128 patients were randomly divided into two groups. In the treatment group of 88 patients, 53 were males and 35 were females, with ages ranging from 38-60 years and averaging 56.1 years. Fifty of these cases were less than 15 days from the onset of stroke, 34 cases were between 16 days to one month, two cases were between 1-2 months, and two cases were between 2-3 months. In the comparison group of 40 patients, 24 were males and 16 were females, with ages ranging from 36-71 years and averaging 55.6 years. Twenty-one of these cases were within 15 days of the onset of stroke, 15 cases were between 16 days to one month, three cases were between 1-2 months, and one case was between 2-3 months. Therefore, there were no significant statistical differences between these two groups in terms of sex, age, and duration of the disease (P>0.05).

Routine Western medical neurological treatment was given to all members of both groups as a basis. In the treatment group, electro-acupuncture and rehabilitation therapy were added. Electro-acupuncture consisted of needling *Lian Quan* (CV 23), *Ren Ying* (St 9) on both sides, the *Hua Tuo* paravertebral points (M-BW-35) on the neck, mouth, tongue, pharynx and motor areas on both sides of the scalp. The needles were manipulated with even supplementing-even draining hand technique. After obtaining the qi, *Lian Quan* and *Ren Ying* were connected to the positive electrodes, and the other points to the negative electrodes. A G6805 electro-acupuncture device was used and set at continuous waves and 150Hz frequency. Treatment was given once per day and lasted 20 minutes each time. Ten treatments equaled one course of therapy, and three courses were administered.

Rehabilitation therapy consisted of psychological counseling, selection of therapeutic environment and body position, bodily function therapy, motor skill enhancement, and direct training. In terms of psychological counseling, the nature of the illness was explained to each patient to help him or her build confidence in the fight for recovery and to reduce anxiety and resistance to treatment. This psychological component positively complemented the physical treatment. Selection of therapeutic environment and body position meant that a quiet, comfortable environment was chosen to avoid disturbance during treatment sessions and meals. When lying down, the patient's body was at an angle of 30-60 degrees to the bed, with his or her neck bending forward. This angle was gradually increased until the patient reached a 90 degree sitting position.

Bodily function therapy consisted of neck exercises, breathing exercises, shoulder exercises, mouth and tongue exercises, speech therapy, and empty swallowing training. Motor skill enhancement consisted of stimulation and massage of the neck and face and massage of the membranes of the pharynx using an ice cube.
Direct training consisted of using different types of food and varying body positions. The patients went through the above prescribed regimen in a measured progression, seeking gradual improvement. This regimen was done once a day, lasting 30 minutes

each session. Ten days equaled one course of treatment and three courses were administered.

The degree of difficulty swallowing was assessed before and after treatment using a point system: Basically cured meant that the patient scored nine or more points. Improved meant a score of 3-8 points. No effect meant a score of 1-3 points. The following table shows the results of the two groups.

Comparison between the two groups showed a remarkable difference (P< 0.01). The treatment group had better results in both their cure rate and total effectiveness. According to the authors of this study, the combination of therapies for post-stroke difficulty swallowing greatly shortened the recovery period and prevented or reduced the occurrence of complications in the patients in the treatment group. The patients' nutritional status improved and their confidence was boosted. During rehabilitation therapy, it was crucial to be able to accurately assess the patients' ability to swallow in order to avoid erratic swallowing. It was equally important to be prepared to perform emergency intervention when necessary.

In the second clinical trial, Dr. Luo Weiping and associates from the Department of Rehabilitation of Zhongshan Chinese Medical Hospital studied the effects of acupuncture combined with physical thera-py on difficulty swallowing.[9] All patients enrolled in this study had an established diagnosis of CVA using CT scan or MRI. All had either hemorrhagic or ischemic stroke complicated by difficulty swallowing. All were also within six months of the onset of stroke and were classified in TCM as channel and network vessel stroke victims. These patients ages ranged from 15-70 years. Patients with poor overall health, with severe disease of the heart, lungs, liver, or kidneys were excluded. Also excluded were those with severe cognitive impairment or with no desire to go through physical therapy. Sixty hospitalized patients who met the foregoing criteria were randomly and equally divided into two groups. The treatment group was treated with acupuncture combined with swallowing training. The comparison group was only treated with swallowing training. There was no significant statistical difference between the two groups in their overall medical and general conditions (P>0.05).

In the treatment group, the main acupoints selected were mostly on the neck. These consisted of *Feng Fu* (GV16), *Feng Chi* (GB 20), *Yi Feng* (TB17), *Wan Gu* (GB12), *Yi Ming* (M-HN-13), *Tian Tu* (CV 22), *Ren Ying* (St 9), and *Lian Quan* (CV 23). Extra-channel points included *Wai Jin Jin* located one inch to the left side and one inch lateral to the upper border of the hyoid bone, *Wai Yu Yue* located one inch to the right side and one inch lateral to the upper border of the hyoid bone; Glossopharyngeal Point located

	Number	Basically Cured	Improved	No Effect	Total Effectiveness (%)
Treatment Group	88	23	49	16	81.82
Comparison Group	40	3	22	15	62.50

Table 5. Comparison of Efficacy between the 2 Difficulty/Swallowing Groups

in the depression 0.5 inches lateral to the midline of hyoid bone and the Adam's apple; and Levator Pharynx Point located anterior and inferior to the mastoid process along the posterior border of the mandible. Points on the face included *Di Cang* (St 4), *Jia Che* (St 6), *Shui Gou* (GV 26), and *Cheng Jiang* (CV 24). Scalp points included the lower 1/3 portion of the Motor Area. In addition, auxiliary points were selected based on TCM pattern discrimination. *Tai Chong* (Liv 3) and *Zu Lin Qi* (GB 41) were added for ascendant liver yang hyperactivity. *Zu San Li* (St 36), *Guan Yuan* (CV 4), and *Xue Hai* (Sp 10) with draining technique were added for qi vacuity and blood stasis. *Tai Xi* (Ki 3) and *San Yin Jiao* (Sp 6) with supplementing technique were added for yin vacuity and stirring of wind. For phlegm heat bowel repletion, *Zhi Gou* (TB 6) and *Feng Long* (St 40) with draining technique were added. The direction of insertion at *Feng Chi, Yi Feng, Yi Ming,* and *Wan Gu* was toward the Adam's apple to a depth of approximately 40 millimeters. Twisting and turning supplementing method with small amplitude and high frequency was used to stimulate these points for one minute. At *Tian Tu,* insertion was perpendicular at first. Then the tip of the needle was pointed transversely downward and slowly inserted to the depth of approximately 25-40 millimeters. This needle was immediately withdrawn after the arrival of qi.[10]

Perpendicular insertion was used at the other points on the neck. Needling of these points caused strong sensation spreading to the pharynx. Depending on the pattern discrimination, the stimulation technique applied to the three points on the face was either light supplementing or draining method after obtaining the qi. *Shui Gou* was needled with strong stimulation. The scalp needle was inserted horizontally at an angle of 15 degrees. The depth was 3-4 centimeters, and

the frequency of twisting was 200 times per minute. Stimulation lasted five minutes each time and was repeated three times during each treatment. One acupuncture treatment was administered per day, with the needles retained for 30 minutes. Fourteen days equaled one course of treatment.

Swallowing training was divided into two parts—basic training and food intake training. Basic training involved the training of all swallowing mechanisms, including the mouth, jaw, lips and tongue. Exercises were both active and passive. Jaw exercises included opening and closing the jaws. Lip exercises included closing, opening, and raising the corners of the mouth. Tongue exercises included sticking it out, lateral movements, and raising the tip and the root. These exercises were combined with blowing pieces of paper, blowing a candle flame, smiling, frowning, puffing up the cheeks, relaxing the neck, sucking, raising the throat, cold stimulation of the pharynx, *i.e.,* gentle stimulation of the soft palate, root of the tongue, and oropharynx using a cotton swab soaked with ice water, voice training, breathing training, *i.e.,* inhaling, exhaling, and making noise. This training was done once per day and lasted 30 minutes each time.

Food intake training progressed gradually from semisolid foods, such as fruit popsicles, yogurt, and egg soup, to solid food. The patient would be lying face upward with their body propped up 30 degrees, head bent forward, the paralyzed side supported by a cushion behind the shoulder. Using a small, thin spoon, a therapist would feed the patient starting with 3-4 milliliters per spoonful and gradually increase to the normal quantity of 20 milliliters per spoonful. The therapist would instruct the patient to do empty swallowing, alternate swallowing (after swallowing food each time, the patient did empty swallowing or alternated swallowing food with a small amount of water), sideways swallowing (moving the lower jaw to the left or right before swallowing sideways), swallowing with head down (with neck bent forward as if nodding, simulating empty swallowing). Each patient went through these training steps alternately. These training steps were tailored according to each patient's ability to do them. Three to five training sessions were given each day.

Members of the comparison group only received swallowing training. The method was the same as that of the treatment group. After 28 days of treatment, the outcomes in each group was evaluated.

With input from the medical literature, a point system was created based on the severity of difficulty swallowing. Cured was defined as a score of 9-10 points, marked effect meant a score of 6-8 points, some effect meant a score of 3-5 points, and no effect was defined as a score of 1-2 points. Patients were evaluated using this scoring system both before treatment and after 28 days of treatment. The following table shows the outcomes of the two groups in this study.

As shown below, the treatment group scored higher in the cured, marked effect, and total effectiveness categories. The difference between the two groups was statistically significant (P<0.005). This is a clear indication that acupuncture combined with swallowing training achieves better results than swallowing training alone.

According to the authors of this study, swallowing disorders caused by stroke present symptoms in the throat but have their source in the brain. The acupoints chosen for treatment in this study are located on the neck and have both direct and indirect connections to the brain and the throat. Needling those points reinforces the brain and boosts the marrow, frees the flow of the channels and quickens the vessels. It also disinhibits the throat and opens the orifices. Looking at these effects in terms of Western medicine, acupuncture at these points can adjust the nervous system in such a way that benefits in both directions—excitability and inhibition. Combined with swallowing training, acupuncture can either raise the excitability of the nervous system or suppress abnormal reflexes, resulting in the originally inactive synapses becoming active. Thus new pathways for neurotransmitters are formed, and, through restructuring, old remnants can function in a new way to replace lost functionality. Such regeneration can prevent the atrophy of the muscle group around the throat due to inactivity as well as strengthen the movement of and the massaging effect on the tongue muscle and the chewing muscle group. Overall, this can increase the agility of the swallowing reflex of patients. Consequently, erratic swallowing can be avoided, related

	Number	Cured	Notably Improved	Improved	Unchanged	Total Effectiveness (%)
Treatment Group	30	13	10	3	4	86.6
Comparison Group	30	5	8	9	8	73.4

Table 6. Comparison of Efficacy between the 2 Groups

complications in the lungs can be prevented, and patients can receive adequate nutrition.

Dysphagia during the acute stage of stroke mostly affects the voluntary action at the entrance of the mouth and the throat, and the reflective action from the center of the mouth to the esophagus. Therefore, during swallowing training, a body position must be chosen that is safe and has a compensatory function. Of the 60 cases in this study, no erratic swallowing occurred. The results of this study clearly indicate that acupuncture combined with deglutition training is an effective treatment technique for clinical practice. They also demonstrate the advantage of the integration of Chinese and Western medicines.

7. Aphasia

Aphasia, the partial or total loss of power to articulate speech, is one of the five main symptoms which can occur following stroke. Most practitioners agree that this symptom is harder to treat than paralysis. In order to help practitioners make their treatments more effective, Zhao Bai-xiao compiled several articles addressing approaches being used in China which treat aphasia.[11] According to Dr. Zhao, there are three main approaches used to treat aphasia:

1. Whole body treatment based on TCM. During the acute stage, the main points include *Shui Gou* (GV 26), *Bai Hui* (GV 20), *Yong Quan* (Ki 1), the well points, and/or *Shi Xuan* (M-UE-1). Auxiliary points include *Tai Xi* (Ki 3), *Feng Long* (St 40), *San Yin Jiao* (Sp 6), and *Xing Jian* (Liv 2). During the recovery period, the main points include *Cheng Jiang* (CV 24), *Tong Li* (Ht 5), and *Zhao Hai* (Ki 6), while the auxiliary points include *Jin Jin & Yu Ye* (M-HN-20) and *Hua Tuo's* paravertebral points at T5, T7, T9, T11, and T14.

2. Scalp acupuncture. Scalp acupuncture may be combined with body points, especially in the recovery stage. In that case, the main scalp points are Motor Area[12] and Speech I, II, III, [13] while the auxiliary points are *Zheng Ying* (GB 17) and *Lian Quan* (CV 23).

3. Local stimulation on the tongue. There are several different techniques for stimulating points on the tongue in the treatment of post-stroke aphasia. The first is referred to as Dr. Zhang's technique. Have the patient open their mouth and hold the tip of the tongue with gauze, pulling the tongue out from the mouth. Insert a 28 gauge three inch needle horizontally through the muscle level of the tongue. Using the new extra-channel point named *Yu Men*, start one centimeter from the tip on the paralyzed side of the tongue following the direction of the vein and insert a needle 2.5 inches deep from the tip to the root.[14] Use even supplementing-even draining hand technique until the arrival of the qi. During insertion, the patient should be instructed to forcibly say the word "Ahhhhh." Then the needle is removed. Twelve treatments (presumably one treatment per day) equal one course followed by 3-6 days rest. This technique should be repeated for a total of four courses. Auxiliary points include *Tong Li* (Ht 5) and *Tai Xi* (Ki 3). At *Tong Li*, use a running needle to *Shen Men* (Ht 7).

Dr. Jiao's tapping method consists of using a plum blossom needle to tap from the tip of the tongue along the midline to the taste buds and then stop. Dr. Dong's method is simply to bleed *Jin Jin* and *Yu Ye* (M-HN-20). Dr. Tan's "Turtle Head Searching Technique" consists of tilting the patient's head upward, thus exposing the point *Lian Quan* (CV 23). The needle is inserted with three strong thrusts and then pulled out slowly and gently all at one time. Afterwards, *Zeng Yin* (an extra-channel point located 0.5 inch lateral to *Lian Quan*) is needled.[15] Dr. Ma also uses *Lian Quan* (CV 23) to treat aphasia, however, with crowded needle technique across the throat. Dr. Zhao uses a technique based more on Western medicine than on TCM. He needles on the sympathetic nerve at a point 1.5 centimeters lateral to the Adam's apple. Dr. Lai Xin-sheng from the Guangzhou College of Chinese Medicine and Pharmacology uses three points on the tongue.[16] Dr. Lai calls these the "Three Submandibular Points" and uses them as his main points to treat aphasia instead of the more commonly selected points *Jin Jin* and *Yu Ye* (M-HN-20). They consist of *Lian Quan* (CV 23) and two points one inch bilateral to *Lian Quan*. *Lian Quan* is an intersection point of conception and yin linking vessels. Therefore, Dr. Lai believes it is the best point to treat aphasia. The two lateral points are added to increase the effect of the treatment. Additionally, he also needles *Feng Fu* (GV 16), *Ya Men* (GV 15), *Jia Che* (St 6), *He Gu* (LI 4), *Tai Chong* (Liv 3), *Tong Li* (Ht 5), and scalp Speech Areas as auxiliary points.

The following is a study on the treatment of post-stroke aphasia using the Three Submandibular Points by Dr. Li Jing-liang of the Henan University Huaihe Hospital.[17] In this clinical trial there were 102 cases of post-stroke aphasia diagnosed by MRI. These 102 patients were randomly divided into two groups—a treatment and a comparison group. The treatment group consisted of 68 patients 39-74 years of age with an average age of 60. Forty-two of these patients were diagnosed with infarctions and 26 with hemorrhage. In the comparison group, there were 34 patients 40-72 years old with an average age of 59. Twenty-two

of these patients were diagnosed with infarctions and 12 with hemorrhage.

All members of the treatment group received acupuncture at the Three Submandibular Points, *i.e.*, *Lian Quan* (CV 23) and the two extra-channel points approximately one inch lateral to both sides of *Lian Quan*. They were also needled at the auxiliary points *Tong Li* (Ht 5), *He Gu* (LI 4), and *Tai Xi* (Ki 3). If there was blood stasis, *Xue Hai* (Sp 10) was added. If there was high blood pressure, *Tai Chong* (Liv 3) was added, and, for phlegm, *Feng Long* (St 40) was added. A 32 gauge 50 millimeter 1.5 inch needle was first inserted towards the root of the tongue. After the patient felt distention radiating from the root of the tongue toward the throat, the needle was withdrawn. *Tong Li* and *He Gu* were needled with draining technique and the needles were retained for 20 minutes. This treatment was given once per day, with 12 treatments equaling one course. The patient was allowed rest and was re-evaluated between each successive course of treatment.

Patients in the comparison group were given a liquid form of *Dan Shen* (Radix Salviae Miltiorrhizae) added to 250 milliliters of saline solution in an intravenous drip per day. These patients did not receive any acupuncture. After treatment, all patients in both groups were given 20 minutes of speech therapy per day.

Basic cure was defined as the ability to speak clearly and to answer easily and accurately. Marked effect was defined as the ability to speak smoothly and basically clearly and to answer questions. Some effect was defined as improvement in speech but the speech was still slurred and the patient was slow to answer. No effect meant that there was no improvement.

Based on these criteria, 20 cases (29.41%) in the treatment group were judged cured, 24 cases (35.29%) got a marked effect, 18 cases (26.47%) got some effect, and six cases (8.82%) got no effect. Therefore, the total effectiveness rate in the treatment group was 91.18%. In the comparison group, six cases (17.65%) were cured, eight cases (23.53%) got a marked effect, 12 cases (35.29%) got some effect, and eight cases (23.68%) got no effect. Total effectiveness rate in this group was only 76.47%. Thus, the treatment group had significantly better results (P<0.05).

Acccording to Dr. Li, after a stroke, aphasia results from a combination of heart, spleen, liver, and kidney disharmony but is particularly due to an imbalance of the heart and kidneys. The heart opens into the sprout of the tongue and the kidney channel branches to the tongue through the sides of the throat to the root of the tongue. This imbalance creates wind, fire, and phlegm stagnation which makes the tongue stiff and speech difficult. Adding the body points to the treatment helps clear the heart and kidney channels. Local needles on the conception vessel at *Lian Quan* connects the yin lining vessel and clears phlegm fire to ease the flow of the network vessels in the tongue. Strong stimulation clears all of these. Results from the Three Submandibular Points technique for aphasia suggest that this method is effective, quick, economical, and safe.

8. Ataxia

Apoplectic ataxia is a disease related to the blood vessels of the brain. It is a particularly common complication of diseases of the cerebellum and brain stem. In recent years, the success of acupuncture therapy in treating this medical condition has been reported more and more in Chinese medical journals. The following study was reported by Zhang

Yu-lian and associates from the Tianjin College of Chinese Medicine Second Affiliated Hospital.[18] All 102 patients included in this study were hospitalized. They were randomly assigned to the treatment and comparison groups at a ratio of 2:1. Of the 68 subjects in the treatment group, 52 were male and 16 were female. Among them were 28 cases of cerebellum infarction, nine cases of cerebellum hemorrhage, 16 cases of brain stem infarction, seven cases of brain stem hemorrhage, and eight cases of cerebellum stem infarction. Of the 34 subjects in the comparison group, 28 were male, six were female. There were 14 cases of cerebellum infarction, six cases of cerebellum hemorrhage, eight cases of brain stem infarction, three cases of brain stem hemorrhage, and three cases of cerebellum stem infarction. All patients in both groups were between 35-75 years of age and were all diagnosed through CT scan or MRI to have had an infarction or hemorrhage of the cerebellum or the brain stem. The duration of disease was within three months, with ataxia as the main symptom. Those with cognitive impairment, paralysis or with muscle strength below grade V, or severe complications were excluded from this clinical trial.

All members of the treatment group received scalp acupuncture. For improving balance, three needles were located below the occipital protuberance with one needle right at the center and the other two 1.5 inches bilateral to the first insertion. For improving motion, the other three needles were located at 0.5 centimeters in front of *Bai Hui* (GV 20) at a 45 degree angle to a line running anterior and inferior.[19] Points on the neck were *Feng Chi* (GB 20), *Feng Fu* (GV 16), and *Hua Tuo's* paravertebral points at C3, C4, and C5. With the patient in a sitting position, a needle was inserted at a 15 degree angle at the scalp points and quickly pushed in below the subcutaneous layer. Then it was inserted through the galea aponeirotica to a depth of 1.5-1.8 inches. Manipulation was done with nine lifting and six thrusting supplementing and draining technique. Depending on the individual's condition, either the technique of forceful thrusting with slow lifting 9-27 times or that of slow thrusting with forceful lifting 6-18 times was applied. This was followed by fast twisting 30 times, with the amplitude back and forth about 180 degrees at a frequency around 200 times per minute.[20] The depth of the insertion at *Feng Chi* was 1.2-1.5 inches, the tip of the needle directed towards the tip of the nose.[21] At *Feng Fu,* the depth of the insertion was 1-1.2 inches. The tip of the needle was pointing downward and should not point upward.[22] The depth of insertion at C3, C4, and C5 paravertebral points was 1.2 inches. The manipulation on these points was the same as above.

 In the comparison group, the following points were needled: *Bai Hui* (GV 20), *Feng Chi* (GB 20), *Jian Yu* (LI 15), *Qu Chi* (LI 11), *Wai Guan* (TB 5), *He Gu* (LI 4), *Zu San Li* (St 36), *Yang Ling Quan* (GB 34), *Feng Long* (St 40), and *Tai Chong* (Liv 3). Routine procedures and techniques were followed. Needles were retained in both groups for 30 minutes each time, and one treatment was administered per day. Five treatments equaled one course of treatment, patients were given a one-day rest between successive courses. Each group received four courses of treatment.

Based on Fugl-Meyer and Lindmark's balanced point scoring standard, a measurement system for ataxia was created by Zhang Yu-lian *et al.* to evaluate the effectiveness of treatment. A point score was given to each of 13 items related to symptoms of ataxia. Each score ranged from 0-4 points. The maximum total score was 52 and the minimum was zero. Cure was defined as a total score equal to or more than 50 points or an improvement in total score of 30 points or more. Marked effect was defined as an improvement of 20 points or more. Some effect meant an improvement of 10 points or more. No effect meant an improvement of less than 10 points. The following table shows the outcomes of the two groups based on these criteria. These outcomes clearly indicate that the treatment group got better results than the comparison group.

 According to the authors of this study, the main function of the cerebellum is to coordinate and synchronize the activities of muscle groups and to adjust the strength of myotasis during voluntary movement of the body. It also maintains balance of the body. Disease in the cerebellum often leads to widespread loss of smooth coordination in voluntary movement which manifests as ataxia in the trunk and limbs. The cerebellum is linked to the brain stem with the same arterial blood supply from the basilar artery system. Hence diseases of the brain stem also cause cerebellum ataxia. Past

Group	No.	Cure	Marked Effect	Some Effect	No Effect	Total Effect
Treatment	68	24	32	12	0	100%
Comparison	34	2	7	17	8	75%

Table 7. Comparison of Efficacy between the Two Groups

Group	No.	Score Before Treatment	Score After Treatment	P Value
Treatment	68	23.72±1.87	48.24±2.34	<0.01
Comparison	34	26.53±2.07	35.58±1.96	<0.05

Table 8. Comparison of Before and After Scores of the Two Groups

research has shown that stimulation of the scalp can increase blood flow in the cortex area and in corresponding areas that can facilitate the establishment of collateral circulation. This improves blood and oxygen supply to the cortex and speeds up the recovery. Because the cerebellum is closely related to the cerebrum, the effects of needle stimulation of the cortex translate to the brain stem and, in turn, to the cerebellum, which helps recovery from the impairment. In this study of treating post-stroke ataxia, it was discovered that the earlier treatment was started, the better the results. Treatment within two weeks of onset was particularly advantageous and brought good results. This treatment technique is simple, easy to use, and has verifiable efficacy.

9. Muscular Atrophy of the Extremities

Muscular atrophy is a common symptom associated with hemiplegia resulting from stroke. The following is a study comparing two different treatments, the first using an awn needle and the second using filiform needles to treat muscular atrophy.[23] Patients enrolled in this study totaled 98, 66 males and 32 females. Among these, there were 61 cases of cerebral infarction and 37 of hemorrhage. These patients were randomly divided into two groups—a treatment group of 50 patients and a comparison group of 48. There were no significant differences in clinical symptoms between the two groups. They all also suffered from hemiplegia in the extremi-

ties. Prior to stroke, both extremities had basically been balanced. Onset of illness in these patients had occurred within 1-6 months prior to treatment. In addition, the difference in circumference between the healthy and afflicted extremities was more than two centimeters.

All members of the treatment group were treated with 6-8 inch awn needles with a diameter of 0.6 millimeters. Running needle technique was used on the affected side as follows:

Jian Yu (LI 15) ———> *Shou Wu Li* (LI 13)
Shou San Li (LI 10) ———> *Pian Li* (LI 6)
Bi Guan (St 31) ———> *Fu Tu* (St 32)
Zu San Li (St 36) ———> *Xia Ju Xu* (St 39)

After routine sterilization, needles were obliquely inserted at a 45 degree angle. On reaching the subcutaneous fascia, the needle angle was changed to 25 degrees. Needles were lightly manipulated and slowly inserted further until a strong sensation of qi was obtained or even sensory transudation was felt. The needles were retained for 30 minutes per treatment and were extracted slowly to the subcutaneous layer before being quickly withdrawn. Punctured points were covered with transfusion tape to prevent infection. A single channel was used on each extremity per treatment, one for the upper and another for the lower, and each was used alternately.

In the comparison group, all patients were treated with acupuncture using filiform needles. The acupoints used on the affected side were *Jian Yu* (LI 15), *Bi Nao* (LI 14), *Qu Chi* (LI 11), *Shou San Li* (LI 10), *Wai Guan* (TB 5), and *He Gu* (LI 4) for the upper limb, and *Bi Guan* (St 31), *Fu Tu* (St 32), *Zu San Li* (St 36), *Feng Long* (St 40), and *Tai Chong* (Liv 3) for the lower limb.

Treatments were administered once per day for both groups, with 10 treatments equaling one course. Five days of rest followed each course. Evaluation of outcomes was conducted after 45 days of treatment.

Outcomes were divided into effective and ineffective. Effective meant that the difference in circumference between the healthy and affected extremities had reduced by more than two centimeters and that muscle strength and function of affected extremities was significantly improved. Ineffective meant that the difference in circumference between the healthy and affected extremities had reduced by less than two centimeters and that there was no significant recovery of muscle strength or function of affected extremities. Based on these criteria, treatment in 42 cases in the treatment group was effective, while treatment was ineffective in the other eight, for a total effectiveness rate of 84%. In the comparison group, treatment was effective in 29 cases and ineffective in 19, for a total effectiveness rate of 60.4%. Therefore, a significant difference was noted in the outcomes between these two groups (P<0.01). Both groups showed some improvement of muscular atrophy but the treatment group showed significantly more improvement.

According to Dr. Liu, stroke results from counterflow of the qi and blood leading to cerebral infarction or hemorrhage. This counterflow also carries phlegm and fire with it which leak into the channels. Thus the circulation of qi and blood is blocked,

resulting in malnourishment of the muscles and sinews. Muscular atrophy or wilting occur. Contemporary Western medicine believes that muscular or disuse atrophy is due to the loss of motor function. Awn needles have a thicker and longer body. They belong to the big needle category of the nine needles. They are normally inserted horizontally along the channel and pass through several acupoints simultaneously. They produce strong stimulation, quickly obtain the qi, easily achieve sensory transudation, and inflict little pain. In this study, awn needles were modified to be shorter and thinner than usual and their method of insertion was also modified. Awn needling stimulates the circulation of qi in the affected extremity, quickens the blood and transforms stasis, eliminates phlegm, and nourishes the sinews and joints in order to treat atrophy. Supplementing technique was mainly used with a longer needle retention time. Since awn needles cover larger areas of the body, Dr. Liu recommends that they be handled lightly, swiftly, and gently. Strict sterilization is needed to avoid bigger wounds or infection.[24]

10. Muscular Tension of the Extremities

Increased muscular tension of the apoplectic limb interferes with daily activities and thus, the quality of life. In some severe cases, it can lead to muscle pain affecting the patients's sleep. In the following study conducted by Mi Jian-ping and his associate from the Guangdong Provincial Chinese Medical Hospital, there were 37, 20 males and 17 females, with an average age of 65 years and an average disease duration of 27.3 days (15-134 days).[25] The diagnosis in all these patients was established by CT scan or MRI, and it was found that 27 patients had cerebral thrombosis and 10 had cerebral hemorrhage. In addition, 34 patients had hemiplegia and three had quadraplegia. To be included in this study, patients had to be less than 75 years old, clinically stable, with no deformity of the affected limbs and no major heart, lung, kidney, or blood diseases. Based on the Ashworth classification, muscular tone was divided into five grades from normal (grade 0) to limited flexion and extension (grade 4). An ability in daily life (ADL) index was based on Barthel SHIs index. Accordingly, a score of 0-34 points meant that the patient was totally dependent, a score of 35-79 points mean the patient was wheelchair bound and required partial assistance, a score of 80-99 points meant that the patient was self-reliant for most of their daily life activities, and a score of 100 points meant the patient was totally self-reliant.

Acupoints needled included the Motor Area of the cerebral cortex on the scalp, *Ji Quan* (Ht 1), *Shao Hai* (Ht 3), and *Ling Dao* (Ht 4) if the upper extremity was affected, and *Ji Men* (Sp 11), *Qu Quan* (Liv 8), *Xi Quan* (Liv 7), and *Zhong Feng* (Liv 4) if the lower extremity was affected. After successfully obtaining the qi, the needles were connected to a G6805 electro-acupuncture machine which was set at 60-80 Hertz. Each treatment lasted for 30 minutes, and the treatment was given six times per week for five weeks.

In terms of muscular tension, cure was defined as a return to normal in muscular tension. Marked improvement meant that muscular tone had improved two grades or better. Some improvement meant that muscular tone had improved one grade, and no effect meant that there was no obvious improvement in muscular tone or it had worsened. Based on these criteria, one patient was considered cured, 14 patients experienced a marked improvement, and 10 patients experienced some improvement.

Therefore, the total effectiveness rate in terms of muscular tension was 83.8%. As for improvements in activities of daily living, marked improvement meant that the ADL index improved 20 points or more with a total of more than 60 points. Some improvement meant that the ADL index improved 10-19 points with a total of 41-60 points. No improvement meant that the ADL index improved less than 10 points with a total of less than 40 points. Based on these criteria, 14 patients registered marked improvement in their ADL and 18 patients experienced some improvement. Thus the total effective rate for improvement in ADL was 86.5%.

According to Dr. Mi, increased muscle tension is a manifestation of stirring of internal wind. This stirring of internal wind damages the liver which in turn affects the sinews, resulting in increased muscular tension or contraction. In Chinese medicine, it is also believed that yin vacuity includes blood vacuity resulting in malnourishment of the sinews. Therefore, the above protocol addressed these disease mechanisms by moving the qi and quickening the blood with electro-acupuncture at points of the heart channel for the upper limb and the liver channel for the lower limb on the affected side. The authors concluded that the electro-acupuncture employed in this study was simple, inexpensive, and highly effective for the relief of increased muscular tension of the extremities after a stroke.

11. Disturbances in Mental Ability

Jiang Dong-xiang *et al.* from the China-Japan Friendship Hospital reported that the external application of selected Chinese herbal medicines to appropriate acupoints has a definite curative effect on mental disturbance arising from diseases of cerebral blood vessels.[26] The 65 subjects in this study were all patients with cerebral blood vessel disease who had been hospitalized. Among them, there were 51 males and 14 females aged 48-81 years, with an average of 62 years. All these patients were diagnosed by CT scan. There were 42 cases of cerebral infarction and 23 cases of cerebral hemorrhage, all with a duration of disease of less than six months. All cases exhibited disturbance of mental activity. Patients' ability to compute, remember, and orient themselves were all low, scoring less than or equal to class III according to the Standard Mentality Disturbance Assessment Method. These patients were randomly divided into a treatment group and a comparison group. Of the 34 patients in the treatment group, 20 were low in all three abilities, nine were low in two abilities, and five were low in one ability. Of the 31 patients in the comparison group, 18 were low in all three abilities, seven were low in two abilities, and six were low in one ability.

The following scoring system was created to assess the ability to do computations:

Class 0: No ability to compute = 0 points
Class I: Able to count from 1 to 10 = 20 points
Class II: Able to do accurately single digit addition = 40 points
Class III: Able to do accurately single digit addition and subtraction = 60 points
Class IV: Able to do accurately two-digit addition and single digit subtraction = 80 points
Class V: Normal computation ability = 100 points

Ability to remember was graded and scored as follows:

Class 0: No ability to remember = 0 points
Class I: 20 points

Class II: 40 points
Class III: 60 points
Class IV: 80 points
Class V: 100 points

Points were scored according to each patient's answers to two groups of questions. Group 1 questions included the following: "Did you have any discomfort prior to the cerebral disease?" "Were there any major events in China in 1976?" "When were you married, year and month?" "In what year was the People's Republic of China founded?" "When did you start elementary school?" Each correct answer was worth 10 points. As for the group 2 questions, each patient was presented with and asked to recognize and commit to memory five objects. Five minutes later, the patient was asked to recall the five objects. Each correct recall was worth 10 points.

Cognitive ability was scored as follows:
Class 0: No cognitive ability = 0 points
Class I: 20 points
Class II: 40 points
Class III: 60 points
Class IV: 80 points
Class V: 100 points

Points were scored according to each patient's answers to five questions. Each correct answer was worth 20 points. The questions consisted of: "Is it morning or afternoon now (or day or night, winter or summer)?" "Where are you now?" What is the name of this item (used in daily life)?" "What is the name of the job title of a medical staff member wearing a uniform?" "Which is the patient's left hand and right hand?"

All members of the treatment group were treated with heated Chinese medicinals applied to acupoints. The herbal formula which was meant to supplement the qi and transform stasis consisted of: *Huang Qi* (Radix Astragali), 60g, *Wei Ling Xian* (Radix Clematidis), 60g, *Lu Jiao Shuang* (Cornu Degelatinum Cervi), 60g, *Chi Shao* (Radix Paeoniae Rubrae), 20g, *Chuan Xiong* (Rhizoma Chuanxiong), 30g, *Hu Zhang* (Rhizoma Polygoni Cuspidati), 30g. These medicinals were mixed together and made into an alcohol extract. Then the volatile oils of *Ding Xiang* (Fructus Caryophylli) and *Rou Gui* (Cortex Cinnamomi) were added to the extract. After removal of the alcohol, the mixture became an emulsion which was stored in a refrigerator. At the time of treatment, some emulsion was evenly spread on two pieces of 4cm by 4cm gauze and placed on *Qi Hai* (CV 6) and *Ming Men* (GV 4). An electric heating silk belt was put on top of the gauze pads. Treatment was applied once or twice per day with each treatment lasting for one hour. One course of treatment consisted of two weeks of therapy, and the patients in this group were given 2-4 courses of treatment. The authors of this article reported having no contraindication to using this method.

Members of the comparison group were given routine treatment using Chinese medicinals taken orally. The herbal formula *Bu Qi Hua Yu Tang* (Supplement the Qi & Transform Stasis Decoction) consisted of the same medicinals used for the treatment group but the doses were different: *Huang Qi* (Radix Astragali), 40g, *Wei Ling Xian* (Radix Clematidis), 30g, *Lu Jiao Shuang* (Cornu Degelatinum Cervi), 30g, *Chi Shao* (Radix Paeoniae Rubrae), 10g, *Chuan Xiong* (Rhizoma Chuanxiong), 10g, *Hu Zhang* (Rhizoma Polygoni Cuspidati), 15g. These medicinals were slow boiled in water and taken once in the morning and once in the evening each day. Each course of treat-

ment was two weeks long, and 2-4 courses of treatment were administered.

All patients in both groups were also administered *Nao Huo Su* (Brain Activity Simple, an unidentified medicine) added to a 250 milliliter intravenous saline solution once per day. One course of treatment equaled two weeks, and 1-2 courses were given. Occupational therapy was also given to both the treatment and comparison groups during the course of this study.

Cure was defined as the subjective disappearance of symptoms with scores for computation, memory, and cognitive ability all at a class V level. Marked effect was defined as the subjective improvement in symptoms with scores for the three abilities raised by one level for two items or raised by two levels for one item. Some effect was defined as the subjective improvement in symptoms with the score of one of the three abilities raised by one level. No effect meant that there was no improvement in symptoms after treatment and the ability scores were not raised. Based on these criteria, of the 34 cases in the treatment group, five (14.7%) were judged cured, 20 (58.8%) achieved a marked effect, and nine (26.5%) got some effect. Thus the total effectiveness rate was reported as 100%. Of the 31 cases in the comparison group, 13 (41.9%) got a marked effect, 15 (48.4%) got some effect, and three (9.7%) got no effect. The total effectiveness rate in that group was 90.3%. The difference between the two groups was statistically significant (P<0.01), indicating that the efficacy for the treatment group was clearly superior to that of the comparison group.

The table on the next page makes it obvious that the treatment group had a far superior

Compatability	Before		After	
	Treatment Group	Comparison Group	Treatment Group	Comparison Group
Computation	36.08±7.25	35.46±7.13	77.45±10.66	56.95±8.37
Memory	34.12±6.59	34.87±6.81	83.17±10.34	59.17±9.72
Cognitive	35.37±7.14	36.09±7.21	78.12±11.78	58.13±9.45

Table 9. Comparison of Mental Capacity before and after treatment

increase in mental capacity scores compared to the comparison group. This data confirms that the external application of heated Chinese medicinals to acupoints can bring about a greater degree of healing of loss of mental function ability resulting from cerebral vascular disease.

According to the authors of this study, disturbance of mental activity is classified in Chinese medicine as feeble-mindedness. Patients with this condition typically manifest vacuity at the root and repletion in the tips or branches. This means the patient suffers from a vacuity of the five viscera with the weakness of spleen and kidney qi as the main culprit, while blood stasis is the most common pattern or mechanism of repletion. Accordingly, the treatment principles should be to boost the qi and warm the kidneys, thus transforming stasis and freeing the flow of the vessels. The Chinese medicinals used in the above protocol have exactly these therapeutic functions. As for the two acupoints, *Qi Hai* is located on the conception vessel, and *Ming Men* is located on the governing vessel connected to the brain. They intersect through the girdle vessel to strengthen the spleen and kidneys. The method of application enables the medicinal ingredients to penetrate through the skin to enter the respective channels. The addition of heating works as a type of warming moxibustion.

12. Sensory Disturbance

Stroke patients often suffer from varying degrees of sensory disturbance depending on the nature, location, and scope of their disease. Such impairment includes feelings of pain and heat as well as disturbances in tactile feeling on the upper part of the body. There may also be disturbances in one's sense of joint position, the ability to perceive the extent, direction, or weight of movement, and one's ability to feel interior pressure. It may also include impairment of the complex senses of sterognosis, dyschiasia, dysmetria between two points, and circle graphic chart impairment which are all controlled by the cerebral cortex. In the following study, Bai Hui-mei *et al.* describe their use of body acupuncture and scalp needling to treat post-stroke sensory disturbance.[27] The 188 patients included in this study were hospitalized between 1994-2002. There were 98 cases of brain infarction, 64 cases of recovery-phase brain hemorrhage, and 26 cases of post-stroke sequelae in this cohort. Among these were 102 males and 86 females 40-78 years of age. The shortest duration of disease was three hours and the longest was 1.5 years. All these patients had been diagnosed by CT scan or MRI. The locations of the disease were mostly at the lobules parietalis, the posterior branch of the capsula interna, and the thalamus. Most of the patients had accompanying motor impairment, but none had cognitive impairment.

Scalp needling consisted of four lines. The first line ran from *Bai Hui* (GV 20) to *Qian Ding* (GV 21). The second line ran from *Cheng Ling* (GB 18) to *Zheng Ying* (GB 17). The third line ran from *Bai Hui* (GV 20) at a 45 degree angle anterior and obliquely for 1.5 inches, while the fourth line ran from *Cheng Ling* (GV 18) at a 45 degree angle exterior and inferior for 1.5 inches. Body acupoints consisted of *Feng Chi* (GB 20), *Jian Yu* (LI 15), *Qu Chi* (LI 11), *Wai Guan* (TB 5), *Si Jiang*,[28] *Zu San Li* (St 36), and *Yong Quan* (Ki 1). Scalp points were needled from superior to inferior and from posterior to anterior transdermally using lifting and thrusting hand technique. The depth of insertion was small but the amplitude of manipulation was large. Needles were stimulated on both sides of the head at the same time for 30 seconds each. Treatment was administered twice per day, needling the affected side in the morning and the opposite side in the afternoon. In terms of body needles, after the arrival of the qi subsequent to insertion, lifting and thrusting, and twirling hand techniques were used for 15 seconds per point, with the needles being retained for 30 minutes. Patients received body acupuncture also twice per day, using the same points and the same techniques in the morning and afternoon. Appropriate Western and/or Chinese medicines were prescribed during hospitalization to deal with complications as indicated.

To assess the outcomes of this study, the traditional nonquantitative method for neurological examination was used, and all patients received a battery of sensory tests for pain, heat, position of joints, sensitivity to pressure, etc. Cure was defined as an absence of any overly sensitive sensory input and an accurate sense of proportion for all tested items. Marked effect was defined as improvement in overly sensitive sensory input and an accurate sense of proportion on 5-6 items tested. Some effect was defined as improvement in overly sensitive sensory input and an accurate sense of proportion on 3-4 items tested. No effect was defined as no improvement in overly sensitive sensory input and an accurate sense of proportion in only 1-2 items tested.

Based on these criteria, 88 cases (47%) were cured, 64 cases (34%) got a marked effect, 28 cases (15%) got some effect, and eight cases (4%) got no effect. Thus the total effectiveness rate was 96%. Of the eight cases that experienced no effect, four had a disease duration of more than one year and had also had unsuccessful treatment with Chinese and Western medicine prior to this study. The other four patients had large-sized infarcts in the capsula interna area. There were also mean improvements in high and low shear, whole blood viscosity, plasma viscosity, and hematocrit, erythrocyte aggregation index, ESR, and fibrinogen. Similarly, there were also significant mean improvements in the blood flow rates in the basal artery network from before to after treatment.

According to the Chinese authors of this study, the method of harmonizing the spirit and quickening the network vessels using acupuncture was the innovation of Professor Guo En-ji. This method combines scalp acupuncture with body acupuncture. According to this methodology, stroke is categorized as impediment of the brain and its vessels with disharmony of the spirit and mind. Hence scalp acupuncture is used for harmonizing the spirit and mind and quickening the network vessels, while body acupuncture is used to improve the handicapped function of the limbs by freeing the flow of the channels and quickening the network vessels.

13. Shoulder Pain

Shoulder pain on the paralyzed side is a common sequela of stroke which is seen in up to 84% of stroke victims. This condition not only affects the function of the arm, thus interfering with self-care, it may also affect patient's balance and walking and expose the patient to the risk of falling. It may also eventually lead to muscle contraction and atrophy of the affected limb. The following four studies describes the acupuncture and moxibustion in the treatment of this complication. According to Deng Gai-ying and associates of Guangxi College of Chinese Medicine, stroke is the result of an imbalance in yin and yang as well as a disturbance in the qi and blood which give rise to inflammation, impaired circulation, and contraction of the soft tissues and the muscles around the shoulder resulting in shoulder pain.[29] Therefore, these researchers used acupuncture to rectify and regulate the qi and blood of the affected channels and free the flow of impedient in order to re-establish the normal flow of the qi and blood. Ninety patients whose diagnoses were confirmed by CT scan and MRI were divided equally into

three groups for this study. All patients were mentally clear in patients who had no history of injury and/or arthritis in the affected limb. Their sensory functions were intact. Group A consisted of 30 patients who received acupuncture treatment. Group B consisted of 30 patients who received both acupuncture and medication, and group C consisted of 30 patients who received only medication. The following table shows the demographics of these three groups. There was no significant statistical difference between these three groups in terms of the above parameters (P > 0.05).

All members of group A received acupuncture at *Shui Gou* (GV 26), *Nei Guan* (Per 6), *Tong Li* (Ht 5), *Ji Quan* (Ht 1), *Zu San Li* (St 36), *Xuan Zhong* (GB 39), *San Yin Jiao* (Sp 6), and *Yong Quan* (Ki 1). In addition, auxiliary points were also needled depending on the affected channel. On the hand yang ming channel, *Qu Chi* (LI 11) and *Jian Yu* (LI 15) were needled. On the hand shao yang channel, *Wai Guan* (TB 5) and *Jian Liao* (TB 14) were needled. On the hand *tai yang* channel, *Jian Zhen* (SI 9) and *Hou Xi* (SI 3) were needled, and on the hand *tai yin* channel, *Lei Que* (Lu 7) and *Jian Qian* (M-UE-48) were needled. Patients with vacuity and/or cold symptoms also received warm moxibustion on *Guan Yuan* (CV 4) and *Zu San Li* (St 36). Even supplementing-even draining hand tech-

	Group A	Group B	Group C
Male/Female	18/12	22/8	19/11
Age Range (Average)	40-70 (54)	40-75 (53)	40-78 (51)
Duration of Illness (Days)	12-129	11-155	14-151
Hemorrhage/Thrombosis	20/10	4/16	8/12
Affected Side-Left/Right	17/13	15/15	9/11
Visual Analogue Scale (VAS)	6.27±1.84	6.13±2	6.0±1.84

Table 10. Demographics of the three groups of patients

nique was used. *Shui Gou* was stimulated until there were tears in the patients eyes. *Ji Quan, Nei Guan*, and *San Yin Jiao* were stimulated until there was tingling and/or numbness in the tips of the fingers and toes. After obtaining the qi, the needles were retained for 30 minutes, except at *Ji Quan* at which the needle was withdrawn immediately. The other needles were twisted every 10 minutes. Acupuncture treatment was given once a day, five days per week for four weeks.

In group B, in addition to the acupuncture treatment described above, Chinese medicinals were also administered based on each patient's TCM pattern discrimination. Western medicines were also given to patients with increased intracranial pressure or cerebral edema. Cerebral cell growth factor in a 0.9% sodium chloride solution was prescribed for cerebral nutrition, while fluids and electrolyte balance were treated and maintained as needed. Patients in group C received the same medications as those in group B but no acupuncture. All patients were evaluated on the 30th day of the treatment.

Patients were evaluated for their shoulder pain using the VAS system both before and after treatment. According to the VAS scale for assessing pain, 0-2 equals excellent, 3-5 equals good, 6-8 is fair, and more than eight was poor. The mean VAS scores post-treatment were compared among the three groups. In group A, the mean score was

3.17 ± 1.72. In group B, the mean score was 3.10 ± 1.71, and in group C, the mean score was 5.00 ± 2.30. While there was no significant difference in VAS scores between groups A and B ($P > 0.05$), the VAS scores in these two groups were better than group C ($P < 0.01$) which received no acupuncture. Therefore, there were more patients with excellent and good results after treatment in both groups A and B than in group C. The following table shows the outcomes of individual patients.

The duration of stroke was also analyzed in group A patients' who received acupuncture treatment. It was noted that patients diseased for less than three months responded better than those whose disease had lasted 3-6 months ($P < 0.05$). Hence this study demonstrated that acupuncture treatment, especially for those in the early phase following the stroke, was effective for improving shoulder pain and shortening the duration of this complication.

In the second study, there were 33 males and 23 females aged 41-79 years.[30] The onset of illness had occurred from three days to two years before the beginning of this study.

Depending on which channels traversing the painful shoulder were affected, the corresponding stream point(s) was/were selected for treatment. *Tai Yuan* (Lu 9) was chosen if the pain was located along the hand tai yin channel. *San Jian* (LI 3) was

Group	Excellent (1)	Good (2)	Fair (3)	Poor (4)	(1)+(2)%
A	12	15	3	0	90.0
B	12	16	2	0	93.3
C	4	10	14	2	46.7

Table 11. Outcomes of individual patients

chosen if the pain was located along the hand yang ming channel. *Zhong Zhu* (TB 3) was chosen if the pain was located along the hand shao yang channel, and *Hou Xi* (SI 3) was chosen if the pain was located on the hand tai yang channel. If the pain was found on two or more channels, the stream points of those two or more channels were selected. Forty millimeter fili-form needles were inserted using regular sterilization. When *Tai Yuan* was needled, care was taken to avoid the radial artery. The tip of the needle was pointed upward to a depth of 0.5-1 inches. At *San Jian* and *Zhong Zhu*, the needle tip was also pointed upward to a depth of 1-1.2 inches. At *Hou Xi*, the needle tip was pointed towards *He Gu* (LI 4) to a depth of 1-1.2 inches. When the qi arrived at the shoulder, the practi-tioner manipulated the needles using drain-ing method. The needles were retained in the body for 30 minutes. Acupuncture was performed once per day, with seven treat-ments regarded as one course.

During treatment, passive range of motion (PROM) was performed on the paralyzed shoulder. With the patient lying in a hori-zontal position, the practitioner supported the patient's scapula on the paralyzed side with one hand and their forearm with the other hand. The patient's forearm was flexed toward his/her head starting from a slight angle. The angle was gradually increased, depending on the patient's ability to tolerate pain. The frequency of flexion was 20 times per minute performed throughout the needle retention time. After 1-3 courses of treatment, 52 cases (93%) were cured, three cases (5%) got a marked effect, and one case (2%) got some effect. Therefore, the total effectiveness rate was 100%. The stream points were chosen for this protocol because the author of the *Nan Jing (Classic of Difficulties)* stated, "The

stream [points] govern joint pain."

In the third study,[31] there were 26 males and 21 females 42-89 years of age, with an average age of 65.5 years. These patients had suffered their strokes 1-6 months prior to commencing this study. Twenty-seven of these cases had suffered cerebral infarction, 15 cases had had hemorrhage, and five cases had had external cerebral trauma. The left shoulder was afflicted in 32 cases and the right shoulder in 15 cases. All these cases were diagnosed by CT scan or MRI.

Points were selected according to pathways of the affected channels. *Yu Ji* (Lu 10) was selected for anterior shoulder pain, *He Gu* (LI 4) for top of the shoulder pain, and *Hou Xi* (SI 3) for posterior shoulder pain. Even supplementing-even draining hand tech-nique was used to obtain the qi and direct it to the diseased area. After needling, the patient voluntarily moved his or her upper extremity, moving the affected shoulder joint to the maximum extent. If the patient was unable to voluntarily move their shoul-der and arm, the patient was assisted to do this within tolerable limits. The needles were retained for 30 minutes and manipu-lated every five minutes. Treatment was done once per day, with 10 days equaling one course.

Evaluation was conducted after two such courses. Cured was defined as disappear-ance of pain when the shoulder joint was moved actively or passively. Some effect was defined as a significant reduction in shoulder pain but some pain still present during movement. No effect meant that there was no alleviation of pain or that it got worse. Based on these criteria, 30 cases (63.8%) were judged cured, 12 cases (25.5%) got some effect, and five cases (10.7%) got no effect. Therefore, the total effectiveness rate was 89.3%. According to Dr. Huang, *Yu Ji, He Gu*, and *Hou Xi* were used to free the flow of their respective channels in the affected area.

In the fourth study, there were 17 males and 13 females 42-79 years of age.[32] Onset of illness prior to commencing the treatment described in this study was 1-3 months. The affected upper extremity was moved and the area of most pain was pressed.

Using regular sterilization procedures at the affected areas, needles were inserted to a depth of 0.2 inches, then manipulated in one direction until the needle could not be extracted. Next, a high frequency, light pecking drainage technique was applied for 30 seconds. At the same time, the patient's family member moved the affected shoulder to its maximum ROM, starting from low to maximum pain tolerance. After ROM was completed, a needle was inserted obliquely from four different directions—front, back, left, and right—spaced 1.5 inches away from and pointed toward the area of pain. The patient was required to feel distention in that area. Needles were retained for 30 minutes. After the needles were removed, a family member was asked to administer appropriate range of motion exercises to the affected shoulder. Treatment was done once per day, with 30 treatments equaling one course. Effectiveness was evaluated after two series. Cure was defined as disappearance of shoulder ptosis and muscular atrophy with no apparent pain during movement. Marked effect meant that there was slight shoulder ptosis or lax muscle with slight pain during movement. Some effect meant that there was slight muscle atrophy at the shoulder joint and some shoulder ptosis. However, the pain level was significantly less when compared to the pain prior to treatment. No effect meant that there was no obvious improve-

ment of symptoms. Based on these criteria, four cases were judged cured, 18 cases got a marked effect, seven cases got some effect, and one case got no effect.

According to Dr. Xu, late-stage stroke shoulder pain is due to lack of active or passive movement of the affected extremity. Its TCM causes include constitutional qi and blood vacuity, disharmony among the heart, liver, and kidneys, and engenderment of internal and/or contraction of external evils. These lead to blockage and obstruction of the qi and blood and malnourishment of the muscles and sinews. So-called stuck needling and pecking drainage methods together with range of motion free the flow of the qi and blood and regulate yin and yang. Needling the four corners of an area of pain is able to stimulate the qi and blood over a wide area, while ROM can induce the local qi and increase the circulation of qi and blood. This has both analgesic and strengthening effects on the affected joint. As in so many other of the studies included in this book, it was also observed that the sooner after onset treatment was administered, the quicker the recovery of the extremity.

14. Insomnia

Insomnia is a common complication in post-stroke patients, and poor or insufficient sleep can adversely affect the overall healing process. In the following study, Cai Lang from Dong Zhi Hospital affiliated with Beijing Chinese Medicine University has treated this symptom using the methods of harmonizing the liver and quieting the spirit with acupuncture.[33] Of the 45 cases included in this study, 27 were male and 18 were female. These patients' ages ranged from 48-85 years old, with an average age of 69. The onset of stroke was within three months in 29 cases, within six months in 13 cases, and within two years in three cases. Stroke was caused from infarction in 33 cases, hemorrhage in 10 cases, and from embolism in two cases.

The main points were *Shen Ting* (GV 24), *Nei Guan* (Per 6), *Tai Chong* (Liv 3), *San Yin Jiao* (Sp 6), and *Si Shen Chong* (M-HN-1). Auxiliary points were added depending on TCM pattern discrimination. For internal stirring of wind, *Feng Chi* (GB 20) and *Feng Fu* (GV 16) were added. For phlegm exuberance internally, *Zhong Wan* (CV 12) and *Tian Shu* (St 25) were added. For yin vacuity with fire flaming, *Tai Xi* (Ki 3) and *Xia Xi* (GB 43) were added. For heart-spleen dual vacuity, *Xin Shu* (Bl 15), *Zu San Li* (St 36), and *Qi Hai* (CV 6) were added. After insertion at these points, the needles were retained for 30 minutes. Patients were treated once per day, with 10 treatments equaling one course.

Results were analyzed after two courses. Marked effect was defined as the ability to sleep soundly for six hours after treatment. Improvement was defined as the ability to sleep 4-5 hours but not necessarily every night. No effect meant that there was no improvement in sleep. Based on these criteria, 19 cases (42%) got a marked effect, 22 cases (48.9%) improved, and four cases (8.9%) got no effect.

15. Hypertension

During the post-stroke recovery period, high blood pressure often recurs and threatens the causation of another stroke. In the following study by Chen Song-quan, 36 cases of hypertension in patients during their post-stroke recovery period were treated by acupuncture at the Hangzhou City Red Cross Hospital.[34]

Altogether, there were 66 patients enrolled

in this two-wing comparison study. The acupuncture treatment group consisted of 36 cases, 20 males and 16 females. The ages in this group ranged from 50-85 years old. Twenty-five of these cases were between 2-7 months post-stroke and 11 were 7-20 months. There were four cases of hemorrhagic stroke and 32 cases of ischemic stroke. Overall, the history of hypertension was between 5-12 years. The comparison group consisted of 30 cases, 18 males and 12 females whose ages ranged from 54-82 years. There were 21 cases whose duration of stroke was between 2.5-6 months and nine cases between 7-25 months. There were also three cases of hemorrhagic stroke, and 27 cases of ischemic stroke. Overall history of hypertension was between 3-10 years.

Acupuncture was the main treatment modality in the treatment group. No blood pressure lowering drugs were used. These 36 patients were divided into two subgroups depending on pattern discrimination. Those exhibiting a pattern of heart-spleen-kidney vacuity presented with poor sleep accompanied by dizziness, fatigue, a pale tongue, and a weak pulse. Acupoints selected consisted of *Feng Chi* (GB 20), *Shen Shu* (Bl 23), and *Zu San Li* (St 36). Filiform needles 0.35mm x 50mm long were used along with twirling and even supplementing-even draining hand technique. These needles were retained for 15 minutes each treatment. For patients with yang vacuity, warm moxibustion using moxa rolls or poles were added at the points for five minutes each treatment. Patients with ascendant liver yang hyperactivity presented with vertigo, restlessness, insomnia, a red tongue with slimy fur, and a bowstring pulse. Acupoints selected for those exhibiting this pattern were *Tai Chong* (Liv 3), *Yin Ling Quan* (Sp 9), *Nei Guan* (Per 6), and *Yin*

Group	Cases	Marked Effect	Some Effect	No Effect	P
Treatment	36	24(67%)	11(30%)	1(3%)	<0.05
Comparison	30	14(47%)	12(40%)	4(13%)	<0.05

Table 12. Comparison of results of the Two Groups

Tang (M-HN-3). Using the same size filiform needles, these were stimulated with a combination of twirling and lifting, and thrusting and draining hand technique. The needles were also retained for 15 minutes per treatment. Acupuncture was administered once every other day in both subgroups. Fifteen minutes after each acupuncture session, blood pressure was measured. Ten acupuncture treatments equaled one course of treatment. After each course, a 10 day rest was allowed, after which the next course would start.

In the comparison group, standard blood pressure lowering drugs were used together with other appropriate treatments. No acupuncture was administered and blood pressure was measured weekly.

Marked effect was defined as normal diastolic pressure or improved by two kPa after three months of treatment.[35] In addition, at least one clinical symptom disappeared or two clinical symptoms improved. Some effect meant that the diastolic pressure was still high but was 1-2 kPa lower compared to before treatment. There was also some improvement in the patient's clinical symptoms. No effect meant that neither of the two preceding criteria were met. For patients whose blood pressure returned to normal for three months, follow-up monitoring of their blood pressure was provided for an additional three months. Their condition was judged to be stable if the number of normal results was

greater than 2/3 the total number of checks, the amplitude of fluctuation of the systolic pressure was less than 14 kPa, and their systolic pressure was not more than two kPa above the normal limit for their age. During follow-up observation, those with average diastolic pressure not exceeding 13 kPa were judged to be normal. The table above shows the outcomes based on the above criteria.

Among the 16 patients in the treatment group who received follow-up observation, the stability rate was 75% and the normal rate was 69%. For the 10 patients in the comparison group who received follow-up observation, the stability rate was 60%, and the normal rate was 50%.

According to Dr. Chen, after a stroke patient is stabilized, the patient's blood pressure often fluctuates or remains high. This is a crucial time for the prevention of another stroke. Based on pattern discrimination, such patients usually present with an imbalance of yin and yang, and vacuity and repletion of the liver, kidneys, heart, conception vessel, and *chong mai*. In general, high blood pressure after stroke is typically due to a root vacuity and tip or branch repletion. Hence, it is important to treat both root and branches at the same time. Attempting to quickly lower blood pressure while failing to prevent the underlying causes of blood pressure fluctuation can cause complications. Therefore, while treating any post-stroke sequelae, one must persist in monitoring the blood pressure and strive to achieve its stability. In this study, there was no recurrence of stroke in the treatment group of 36 cases. In the comparison group, the stability rate was lower and there were two recurrences of stroke. Additionally, those patients who suffered side effects from blood pressure lowering drugs soon were rid of those side effects after they switched to acupuncture. At the same time, their clinical symptoms improved.

16. Headache

Zheng Shen-yan and associates from various hospitals affiliated with the Heilongjiang Chinese Medicine University found that stroke patients who suffered from cerebral infarction often complained of headaches which varied in degrees of intensity.[36] Some of these headaches could not be relieved by dehydration and cranial depressurization, thus causing these researchers to conclude these types of headaches were not related to cranial hypertension. Instead, they were due to the acute cranial vascular occlusion which led to compensatory dilatation of extra-cranial vessels. In such cases, bleeding the well points often resulted in immediate relief.

In the following study, there were 30 stroke patients who suffered from cranial infarction. Among these, 19 were male and 11 were female. These patients' ages ranged from 42-78 years. The shortest duration since the onset of stroke was three hours and the longest was five days. All patients suffered from headaches. Mental capacity was clear without significant aphasia. All patients were diagnosed by CT scan.

All these patients were treated with regular dehydration, dissolution, vasodilation, etc. along with bleeding the well points of the unaffected limb: *Shao Ze* (SI 1), *Guan Chong* (TB 1), *Shang Yang* (LI 1), *Zhi Yin* (Bl 67), *Qiao Yin* (GB 44), and *Li Dui* (St 45). Twenty-eight gauge one inch needles were used with a quick blood-letting technique at the above six acupoints, allowing several drops of blood to be squeezed out.

Cure was defined as disappearance of headache within 30 minutes after the bleeding with the effect lasting for more than 24 hours. Some effect was defined as alleviation or disappearance of headache within 30 minutes after bleeding. However, the effect lasted for less than 24 hours. No effect meant that there was no obvious relief of headache within 30 minutes after treatment. Based on these criteria, eight cases were cured, 19 cases got some effect, and three cases got no effect. The total effectiveness rate was 90%.

According to the authors, acute cerebral infarction is categorized as wind stroke in TCM. It is caused by kidney vacuity due to old age with water not nourishing wood. Thus internal wind is stirred, phlegm and fire develop internally, and wind and phlegm leak into channels and network vessels blocking the orifices. Since the channels and network vessels are not freely flowing and the orifices have lost their function, headaches result. Both hand and foot yang channels run to the head. Therefore, acupoints from the yang channels were selected. Well points from the limbs were bled based on the theory of selecting points below for diseases above. Besides, well points are located near where yin and yang connect. Therefore, using well points can free the flow of the channels and network vessels, harmonize yin and yang, and open the orifices. Acupoints on the unaffected limbs were selected because of

Group	Cure	Marked Effect	Some Effect	No Effect
Treatment	40 (50%)	22(27.5%)	10 (12.5%)	8(10%)
Comparison	8 (26.7%)	6(20%)	10 (33.3%)	6(20%)

Table 13. Comparison of results of the Two Groups

higher needle sensitivity.

From the point of view of modern Western medicine, headaches from cerebral infarction are a type of vascular headache due to compensatory vascular dilatation. Bleeding the well points may trigger a certain type of neuroendocrine mechanism and regulate vascular contraction and dilation. This mechanism needs further study.

17. Urinary Incontinence

Post-stroke urinary incontinence may cause the patient to lose self-esteem leading to depression. Infection and even bed sores may also develop. Tian Yuan-sheng and associates from the Henan Chinese Medicine Research Institute have reported effective results treating this condition with acupuncture.[37] The following study included 80 post-stroke patients with the symptoms of urinary incontinence. There were 50 males and 30 females ranging from 36-78 years of age. Forty-two of these patients were within six months of the onset of stroke, 24 patients were within one year, and 14 patients were over one year. There were also another 30 cases in a comparison group that were treated with needling *Guan Yuan* (CV 4).

After routine sterilization, a needle was inserted horizontally and posteriorly at *Bai Hui* (GV 20) to the depth of 1.5-2.5 inches in all members of the treatment group. The needle was twisted rapidly about 200 times per minute for five minutes, followed by a

five minute break. Twisting was repeated three times. Then the needle was withdrawn. In the comparison group, a needle was inserted at *Guan Yuan* (CV 4) obliquely downward two inches in depth. It was important for the patient to feel the needle sensation traveling to the front of the genital area. The needle was retained for 20 minutes. Treatment in both groups was applied once per day, with 10 treatments equaling one course. Outcomes were analyzed after three courses of treatment. Cure meant that the patient regained the feeling of the urge for urination and could control his or her urination voluntarily. Marked effect meant that patients were basically cured but still had occasional episodes of incontinence. Some effect meant that the patient regained the feeling of the urge to urinate but not consistently. Sometimes they had good control, and sometimes they lost control. No effect meant that, after three courses of treatment, there was no change in the patient's symptoms. The table above shows the outcomes based on these criteria. These results showed that there were big differences between these two groups of patients in terms of cure and marked effects. (P<0.01)

According to Dr. Tian, the governing vessel is the ruler of the yang qi of the whole body. Its upper end is in the brain, while its lower part connects to the bladder channel and then to the bladder. *Bai Hui* means "meeting [point] of one hundred." It is also called "the three yangs and five intersections." Needle stimulation on this point has a resuscitative effect. From the perspective of Western medical anatomy, this point is located above the urination center of the brain. Stimulation from needling *Bai Hui* may awaken this center, resulting in the healing of urinary incontinence.

18. Urinary Retention

Normal urination is a function of the qi mechanism, and the mechanisms of stroke may cause inhibition to the body's qi mechanism as a whole. Thus, urinary retention is yet another possible complication in the aftermath of stroke. Li Hua and associates from the First Affiliated Hospital of the Heilongjiang University of Chinese Medicine have reported on their experience treating post-stroke urinary retention with a combination of very simple moxibustion and massage.[38]

There were 30 patients in this study. A moxa roll or pole was held two centimeters away from *Tai Xi* (Ki 3). This was continued until the patient felt warm and comfortable at this area. Moxibustion on *Tai Xi* was administered alternatively on both feet. The total time of moxibustion was 20 minutes. At the same time, the practitioner placed his or her right hand below the patient's navel and pushed along the conception vessel until the top of the pubic symphysis was reached. This massage was also continued for 20 minutes. Meanwhile, the patient was instructed to act as if he or she was urinating. Ten patients were cured, 15 improved, and five got no effect.

According to the Chinese authors of this study, *Tai Xi* is the source point on the kidney channel, and the source point is where essence and qi of the viscera and bowels enter and exit the channel. *Tai Xi* was treated because it internally connects with the kidneys which govern the opening and clos-

ing of the urinary bladder. The heat from the moxibustion warmed the channels and network vessels, regulated the qi, and restored the opening and closing of the urinary bladder. As a result, urine was able to be excreted. From a Western anatomical point of view, the urinary bladder is situated in the hypogastrium, and the conception vessel runs along the centerline of the hypogastrium. Pushing the conception vessel is able to supplement the kidneys and boost the qi as well as augment qi transformation in the urinary bladder. Thus it also helps urination.

19. Constipation

Just as the elimination of urine is dependent on the qi mechanism, so is the elimination of feces. Thus constipation is also a common condition in stroke patients. Although constipation is not life-threatening in and of itself, in the long run, it may impose a health hazard. Long-term use of laxatives can produce numerous side effects. The following two studies published in China show that acupuncture and its related modalities can successfully treat this condition without harmful side effects. The first study was done by Xu Xiu-ju from Heze City in Shandong Province using seeds pressed on the auricle for the treatment of post-stroke constipation.[39] In this study, there were 46 males and 16 females 50-78 years of age. All suffered from constipation following stroke.

The main auricular points used in all patients were Large Intestine, Small Intestine, Lung, and Triple Burner. According to the symptoms, other points such as Endocrine, Sympathetic, Spleen, Stomach, Abdomen, Liver, etc. were also selected. Black *Wang Bu Liu Xing Zi* (Semen Vaccariae) with a diameter of 1-1.5 millimeters were chosen and soaked in 75% alcohol. These were then dried in the sun. Medical adhesive plasters were cut into 4mm x 4mm squares and the seeds were placed in the center of the plasters. After the ear was cleaned with alcohol, the plasters were placed on the auricular points. Each seed was gently pressed on the points with the thumb and index fingers until either distention, pain, or a warm sensation was felt by the patient. Patients were instructed to massage the auricular points several times a day, 1-2 minutes each time. According to the patient's tolerance level, pressure could be increased, thus resulting in an increase in effectiveness. The plasters were changed once every 3-7 days.

In terms of outcomes, effective meant that the stool was soft and easy to pass without strain and bowel movements occurred once every 1-2 days. Ineffective meant that bowel movements were difficult and strained or that stools were dry and difficult to pass. In addition, bowel movements occurred once every three or more days. Based on these criteria, in 59 cases, treatment was judged effective and, in three cases, it was ineffective. Therefore, the total effectiveness rate was 95.1%.

According to Dr. Xu, this technique is safe, easily taught, and free of side effects or toxicity. This technique may be used on any patient with post-stroke constipation regardless of their presenting TCM pattern.

The second study addresses chronic constipation due to severe stroke. After patients are bed-ridden for a long period of time, their peristalsis function typically weakens. The main symptoms of this are abdominal distention and fullness, decreased frequency of bowel movements, and/or difficulty or straining at bowel movements, and dry stools. Such constipation is due to atony of the colon in turn due to pathologic neurological changes following stroke. In the following study, all subjects were hospitalized

stroke patients diagnosed as having chronic constipation.[40] Among these patients, there were 24 males and 14 females aged 50-75 years. Time from onset of stroke to initiating treatment for constipation was 3-7 days. Thirty-two of these cases suffered from cerebral infarction and six from hemorrhage.

The patients were instructed to lay on their sides. After regular sterilization, awn needles 0.4 millimeters in diameter and 5-7 inches in length were inserted at *Da Chang Shu* (Bl 25) and *Qi Hai Shu* (Bl 24). Guided by tweezers, the needles were rapidly inserted into the skin. Thrusting and lifting manipulations were performed until the needles reached 3-6 inches under the skin. After the patient felt the qi sensation as either distention or electrical shock bilaterally along the lateral abdomen or as a running sensation to the hypogastrium, the practitioner thrust and lifted three times before pulling the needles out. In thin patients, the depth of the insertion was only 3-4 inches, while, if the patient was fleshy, the depth was 4-6 inches.[41] After that, the patients lay in a supine position. *Tian Shu* (St 25), *Zu San Li* (St 36), and *Shang Ju Xu* (St 37) were needled to a depth of three inches. The patients were supposed to feel distention during needle manipulation. After the qi was obtained, the needles were retained in the body for 30 minutes. Acupuncture was administered once per day, and five days were regarded as one course. Analysis of outcomes was done after two such courses.

Cured was defined as disappearance of constipation with bowel movements 1-2 times per day or once every other day without any straining. The quantity of stool passed was medium. Some effect was defined as an improvement in constipation as well as abdominal distention. Stool was passed with straining. The quality of stool was slightly hard. The quantity was medium, with more than 100 grams per day. No effect was defined as no improvement in constipation or abdominal distention. The amount of stool was less than 100 grams, was not easily passed even with straining, and an enema was needed. Based on these criteria, 30 patients (78.9%) were cured, five cases (13.2%) got some effect, and three cases (7.9%) got no effect. Therefore, the total effectiveness rate was 92.1%.

20. Edema

Post-stroke edema is usually worse in the distal parts of the limbs and the temperature of the swollen limb is much lower than that of the healthy side at the same level. After treatment with standard body acupuncture, the strength and function of the limbs may have recovered, but the swelling often does not go down. In such cases, Pang Hong from the Chinese Medicine Research Institute used herbal seeds applied to selected points on the ear.[42]

In this study, there were 32 cases, including 11 males and 21 females 45-73 years of age. Their strokes had occurred from one month to one year prior to acupuncture. All cases met the diagnostic criteria established in the national diagnosis standard in China. Judging from the spinal fluid and CT scan examination, 23 cases were caused by ischemia and nine were from hemorrhage. All patients suffered from motion impairment and had swelling in their limbs.

The corresponding points used on the ear were Heart, Kidney, Subcortex, Sympathetic, Liver, Spleen, Triple Burner, and Occiput. One piece of *Wang Bu Liu Xing* (Semen Vaccariae) was placed on a 0.5 x 0.5 centimeter plaster and applied to each selected ear point on one ear. These seeds were removed every other day and fresh seeds were applied to the opposite ear. The patient

also lightly stimulated the seeds about 20 times with finger pressure each time, repeating 3-5 times daily.

Basically cured meant that the swelling of the limb was gone and there was no pitting on pressure or any feeling of swollen discomfort. Improved meant that the swelling had gone down or only appeared in the afternoon. If finger pressure was applied, there was a shallow depression which was relieved quickly after the finger was taken off. The patient described the limb as looser and more comfortable. Unchanged meant that there was no change in the swelling after treatment. Based on these criteria, seven cases (21.9%) were judged basically cured, 20 cases (62.5%) improved, and five cases (15.6%) remained unchanged. The total effectiveness rate was 84.4%.

According to the Chinese author of this study, selection of Heart, Liver, and Spleen ear points was meant to free the flow of the channels and eliminate dampness. Kidney and Triple Burner points were chosen to regulate the water passageways and help to disperse the swelling. Ear Subcortex was chosen to regulate the function of the brain, while ear Sympathetic was meant to regulate the nervous system. The Heart and Occiput points were chosen to improve the blood flow supplying the brain and benefit circulation.

21. Post-CVA Neuralgia

Neuralgia of the affected limbs is yet another common complication in post-stroke patients, and acupuncture has shown good effects with this type of pain. Zhang Tong and associates from the Affiliated Hospital of the Shandong Chinese Medicine University reported their experience using scalp and body acupuncture.[43]

	Group I	Group II	Group III
Mild	13	10	14
Moderate	12	9	11
Severe	7	10	11

Table 14. Distribution of the patients according to severity

Ninety-seven patients with an established diagnosis of CVA were enrolled in this study. Among these, there were 59 patients with cerebral thrombosis and 38 patients with cerebral hemorrhage. These patients were divided into three treatment groups. Group I consisted of 32 patients with 17 males and 15 females aged 38-82 and an average age of 57 years. Group II consisted of 29 patients with 16 males and 13 females aged 41-78 and an average age of 62 years. Group III consisted of 36 patients with 20 males and 16 females aged 40-81 and an average age of 61 years. The severity of neuralgia was categorized into three levels. Mild meant that the pain was bearable and did not interfere with limb activity and sleep. Moderate meant that the pain limited activity of the paralyzed limbs but did not interfere with sleep. Severe meant that the pain was persistent, unbearable, and interfered with sleep. Passive movement of the affected limb might cause sweating and the face turning pale. The table above shows the distribution of the severity of neuralgia among the three groups.

Scalp acupuncture was performed on all members of group I corresponding to the Motor and Sensory area of the cerebral cortex on the affected side (or opposite the side of the paralyzed limb). A 30 gauge acupuncture needle 1.5-2 inches in length was used with rapid twisting for 2-3 minutes. The needles were then left in place for 5-10 minutes. This treatment was given 1-2 times per day. In group II, body acupuncture was performed at *Jian Yu* (LI 15), *Qu Chi* (LI 11), *He Gu* (LI 4), *Wai Guan* (TB 5), *Huan Tiao* (GB 30), *Zu San Li* (St 36), *Yang Ling Quan* (GB 34), *Jue Gu* (GB 39), and *Kun Lun* (Bl 60) on the paralyzed limb. After insertion, the needles were twisted with wide amplitude and then the needles were withdrawn after 5-10 minutes. Treatment was given 1-2 times per day. Members of group III received a combination of the foregoing two treatments. In other words, they received both scalp and body acupuncture. Treatment was given daily for 10 days as one course in all three groups.

In terms of outcomes, excellent meant that the neuralgia was completely relieved. Some

	Excellent	Some Effect	No Effect	Total Effect
Group I	14	14	4	87.5%
Group II	11	13	5	82.76%
Group III	25	9	2	94.44%

Table 15. Treatment results

effect meant that the neuralgia decreased by one grade or more. No effect meant that the neuralgia remained unchanged from before to after treatment. The previous table shows the outcomes of the three groups based on these criteria.

Based on these results, there was no significant statistical difference in the effectiveness among the three groups. However, the combined use of scalp and body acupuncture achieved higher excellent results than the other groups (P< 0.05). Therefore, Dr. Zhang *et al.* concluded that the combined use of scalp and body acupuncture was superior to scalp or body acupuncture alone. It alleviated or totally eliminated the neuralgia of the paralytic limbs in about two-thirds of the patients.

22. Persistent Phrenospasm

In contemporary Western medicine, phrenospasm is due to stimulation of the diaphragmatic nerves. This in turn leads to spasm of the diaphragm resulting in hiccup. In normal, healthy people, phrenospasm is usually caused by exposure to a cold environment, certain foods and drinks, eating too quickly, or mental stress. Usually, episodes are not long-lasting. However, in seriously sick people, phrenospasm increases the severity of disease and suggests an unfavorable prognosis. Many patients with cerebral vascular disease have phrenospasm after stroke due to damage to the function of the vegetative nervous system. This type of phrenospasm is very persistent, difficult to control, and very challenging to treat. It causes much suffering to patients and even presents a potentially serious threat to their lives.

Since 1996, the author of the following study has treated 62 patients suffering from post-stroke persistent phrenospasm with

acupoint injection combined with oral Chinese herbal medicine.[44] This group of 62 included both inpatients and outpatients. Among them were 42 males and 20 females ranging from 41-83 years of age. Duration of disease ranged from four days to three months. CT scanning identified 48 cases of cerebral infarction and 14 cases of cerebral hemorrhage. Phrenospasm or hiccup appeared after stroke in all these patients.

The medication used for the acupoint injection consisted of a mixture of 1.5 milliliters of anisodamine, three milliliters of vitamin B[1], and three milliliters of vitamin B[6]. With the patient lying on his or her back, routine disinfectants were applied to the acupoints. Then the above mixture was injected into *Zhong Wan* (CV 12), *Nei Guan* (Per 6), and *Zu San Li* (St 36) on both sides, 2.5 milliliters of liquid at each point. One injection was administered each day, and five days equaled one course of treatment. This was combined with the oral administration of *Ding Xiang San* (Caryophyllum Powder) plus *Chuan Xiong* (Rhizoma Chuanxiong). Various other Chinese medicinals were added to this base depending on the patient's individual TCM identification.

Using this protocol, 60 patients were cured, meaning that their phrenospasm disappeared. Twenty patients were cured after one injection, 28 were cured after two injections, 12 were cured after three injections, and two got no effect from the injections. Total effectiveness rate was 96.7%. On follow-up after six months, five patients had had a recurrence of persistent phrenospasm. However they responded to more routine treatment and could again be classified as cured.

According to the Chinese author of this study, injection of anisodamine can relax spasm in the diaphragm muscle, while the vitamin B1 and B6 have nourishing effects on the nerves. Acupoint injection allows the slow absorption of medication in those points, and, through the acupuncture channels, the medication can directly reach the source of the disease. Combining injection therapy with oral medication achieves the objective of dissipating the upward rush of qi and stopping the spasm. According to Chinese medical theory, phrenospasm or hiccup is due to the upward counterflow of qi from the stomach disturbing the lungs. For stroke patients with phrenospasm, additional consideration must be given to blockage and obstruction by blood stasis in the blood vessels. Within the above formula, *Ding Xiang* and *Shi Di* (Calyx Kaki) are used to direct the counterflowing qi downward, while *Chuan Xiong* quickens the blood and regulates the qi. This herbal formula has a dependable effect, with the added benefit of preventing recurrence.

23. Persistent Laughing

Some stroke patients develop uncontrollable laughing which requires special treatment. According to clinical observation, most patients experiencing this symptom are overweight. Thus, they have more phlegm, dampness, and turbidity. This phlegm transforms fire, and the fire disturbs the spirit and mind causing uncontrollable laughing when there is no reason for the patient to laugh.

In the following study, Zhang Hai-ji from the Henan Chinese Medical Hospital treated 11 cases of this condition from July 1988 to December 1997.[45] There were seven males and four females in the study whose ages ranged from 50-69 years. The uncontrollable laughing symptoms were experienced from five days to three years after the onset

of stroke. Each patient had received a head CT scan for actual diagnosis of stroke on their first visit which excluded emotional influences and mental problems as the cause of their symptom of laughter.

Needles 1.5 inches long were inserted bilaterally at *Nei Guan* (Per 6) and *Feng Long* (St 40). The two *Nei Guan* points were connected to a G6805 electrical device for 30 minutes using continuous waves. At *Feng Long,* a large twisting draining technique was applied with repeated stimulation every five minutes. The needles were retained for half an hour each time, and treatment was given daily. Three treatments were considered as one course. This was followed by a day of rest before resuming another course.

Cure was defined as complete disappearance of inappropriate laughing. Marked effect meant that laughing spells occurred less than three times per 24 hours. Some effect meant that laughing spells occurred less than six times per 24 hours. No effect meant that the laughing spells remained unchanged from before to after treatment. Based on these criteria, nine cases (81.80%) were judged cured, one case (9.10%) got a marked effect, and one case (9.10%) got some effect. Therefore, the total effectiveness rate was 100%. The shortest period of treatment to obtain results was only two treatments; the longest was six courses of treatment.

According to the author of this study, satisfactory results were the result of the right combination of acupoints. In Chinese medical theory, overweight patients have lots of phlegm and lots of dampness. Because of this, the cause of stroke in such patients is classified as phlegm damp exuberance and obstruction. This disturbs the spirit governed by the heart and results in uncontrollable laughing. The pericardium as the shell of the heart acts as a substitute to accept any evil qi. Therefore, needling *Nei Guan* can out-thrust the evil qi from the body. The second important set of acupoints in this treatment is *Feng Long*, the network point of the stomach channel which is used to transform phlegm and eliminate dampness. Based on the foregoing study, these two points appear to work well together for this special problem.

Endnotes

[1] Hou Dong-fen *et al.*, "Clinical Observations on the Effects of Electro-acupuncture at *Bai Hui* (GV 20) & *Yin Tang* (M-HN-3) in the Treatment of 30 Cases of Post-stroke Depression," *Zhong Guo Zhen Jiu (Chinese Acupuncture & Moxibustion)*, #8, 1996, p. 23-24

[2] Wang Hai-jian, "Clinical Observations on Acupuncture for the Treatment of Post-stroke Depression," *Zhong Guo Zhen Jiu (Chinese Acupuncture & Moxibustion)*, #8, 2003, p. 442-443

[3] Xie Tu-dun *et al.*, "The Acupuncture Treatment on a Particular Point for Post-stroke Motor Impairment of the Thumb," *Zhong Guo Zhen Jiu (Chinese Acupuncture & Moxibustion)*, #11, 2003, p. 678

[4] Ma Guang-hao *et al.*, "Local Penetration Needling in the Treatment of Dysfunctions of the Wrist & Ankle Joints in Patients with Apoplexy," *Zhong Guo Zhen Jiu (Chinese Acupuncture & Moxibustion)*, #9, 2002, p. 587-589

[5] *Wai Shen Men* is located at the ulna side of *Shen Men* (Ht 7). Its name means "Outside of *Shen Men*."

[6] Liu Zhen-chun, "Dysfunction of Upper Limbs as Sequela of Stroke Treated with T-Shaped Needling," *International Journal of Clinical Acupuncture*, #1, 1995, p. 73-74

[7] Zhang Yu-lian *et al.*, "The Treatment of 36 Post-stroke Dysopsia Patients with Scalp Acupuncture & Four Periocular Acupoints,"

Shang Hai Zhen Jiu Za Zhi (Shanghai Journal of Acupuncture & Moxibustion), #4, 2003, p. 6-7

[8] Zong Tao *et al.*, "The Use of Electro-acupuncture in Conjunction with Rehabilitation Therapy for Difficulty Swallowing Due to Stroke," *Liao Ning Zhong Yi Za Zhi (Liaoning Journal of Chinese Medicine)*, #5, 2003, p. 398

[9] Lu Wei-ping *et al.*, "The Therapeutic Effects of Acupuncture Combined with Swallowing Training on Difficulty Swallowing Due to Apoplexy," *Zhong Guo Zhen Jiu (Chinese Acupuncture & Moxibustion)*, #8, 2004, p. 528-530

[10] Warning: The authors of this article used deep insertion and strong stimulation on the acupoints of the neck. Because of the complex anatomy at these point locations, we urge our readers to *not* practice this technique without the supervision of an experienced practitioner. It is very risky and may cause various complications such as bleeding or damage to the nerves, spine, trachea, etc.

[11] Zhao Bai-xiao, "A Discussion of Recent Articles on Acupuncture Methods for Treating Aphasia," *Zhong Guo Zhen Jiu (Chinese Acupuncture & Moxibustion)*, #4, 1997, p. 251-253

[12] Motor Area: This consists of a line starting from a point 0.5 centimeters posterior to the midpoint of the anterior-posterior midline of the head and stretching diagonally across the juncture between the eyebrow-occipital line and the anterior border of the corner of the temporal hairline.

[13] Speech I Area is located at the lower two-fifths of the Motor Area. Speech II Area is found by drawing a line from the parietal tubercle parallel with the anterior-posterior midline of the head. This area is then a vertical line two centimeters posterior to the former line, three centimeters in length. Speech III Area is a parallel line overlapping the Vertigo and Hearing Areas at the midpoint and continues four centimeters posterior.

[14] Caution: This technique easily causes bleeding, resulting in a swollen tongue. At the worst,

it may even cause difficulty breathing or infection.

[15] *Zeng Yin* is an extra-channel point. Its location is the same as *Pang Lian Quan* (M-HN-24), 0.5 inches lateral to *Lian Quan* (CV 23).

[16] Lai Xin-sheng, "Clinical Application of the Three Tongue Points in Aphasia," *International Journal of Clinical Acupuncture*, #2, 1999, p. 185-187

[17] Li Jing-liang, "Clinical Observations on the Acupuncture Treatment for 68 Cases of Post-stroke Aphasia," *Shang Hai Zhen Jiu Za Zhi (Shanghai Journal of Acupuncture & Moxibustion)*, #10, 2003, p. 5-6

[18] Zhang Yu-lian *et al.*, "A Clinical Study on the Treatment of Apoplectic Ataxia with Scalp & Nape Acupuncture," *Shang Hai Zhen Jiu Za Zhi (Shanghai Journal of Acupuncture & Moxibustion)*, #8, 2003, p. 7-8

[19] The author did not specify on which side of the scalp the needle insertion was to be made, or whether insertion on both sides was needed.

[20] Caution: The author treated patients in the sitting position and used a very forceful and strong manipulative technique for stimulation. Since most post-stroke patients are weak, we must point out the potential risk of the patient fainting during such aggressive treatment.

[21] Caution: Care must be exercised to avoid inserting the needle too deeply, risking puncture of the medulla.

[22] Warning: Avoid an excessively deep insertion on *Feng Fu* (GV 16). Extreme care must be taken to avoid inserting the needle upward into the medulla oblongata where it could cause death.

[23] Liu Guo-qing, "Using Awn Needles to Treat 50 Cases of Muscular Atrophy Due to Stroke Hemiplegia," *Liao Ning Zhong Yi Za Zhi (Liaoning Journal of Chinese Medicine)*, #5, 2003, p. 400-401

[24] Warning: This is a special technique which is not commonly used. It requires skillful hands to perform. Practitioners should not attempt to practice this technique without being taught by

someone with experience or under supervision.

[25] Mi Jian-ping, *et al.*, "Clinical Observations on the Reducing Effect of Yin Channel Electro-acupuncture on Muscular Tension of the Extremities in Apoplectic Hemiplegia," *Shang Hai Zhen Jiu Za Zhi (Shanghai Journal of Acupuncture & Moxibustion)*, #10, 2003, p. 7-8

[26] Jiang Dong-xiang *et al.*, "A Clinical Investigation of the Treatment for Mental Activity Disturbance Due to Cerebral Vascular Disease Using Heated Chinese Herbal Medicine Applied to Acupoints," *Zhong Guo Zhen Jiu (Chinese Acupuncture & Moxibustion)*, #9, 1997, p. 532-534

[27] Bai Hui-mei *et al.*, "Clinical Observations on the 188 Cases of Acupuncture on Sensory Disturbance Due to Apoplexy," *Shang Hai Zhen Jiu Za Zhi (Shanghai Journal of Acupuncture & Moxibustion)*, #10, 2003, p. 3-4

[28] *Si Jiang* is an extra-channel point located 5.5 *cun* above the midline of the patella at the front part of the upper leg.

[29] Deng Gai-ying *et al.*, "The Short-term Therapeutic Effects of Acupuncture & Moxibustion on Shoulder Pain in Patients with Post-stroke Hemiplegia," *Zhong Guo Zhen Jiu (Chinese Acupuncture & Moxibustion)*, #12, 2004, p. 815-817

[30] Dang Du-hua *et al.*, "Needling Mainly on the Stream Points to Treat 56 Cases of Shoulder Pain Due to Hemiplegia," *Shang Hai Zhen Jiu Za Zhi (Shanghai Journal of Acupuncture & Moxibustion)*, #6, 1997, p. 18

[31] Huang Wen-chuan, "Clinical Observations on 47 Cases Using Acupuncture for Hemiplegic Shoulder Pain," *Lin Chuang Zhen Jiu (Clinical Acupuncture & Moxibustion)*, #6, 1997, p. 28

[32] Xu Yu-jue, "Acupuncture in the Treatment of 30 Cases of Late-stage Stroke Shoulder Pain," *Zhong Guo Zhen Jiu (Chinese Acupuncture & Moxibustion)*, #5, 2000, p. 278

[33] Cai Lang, "Harmonizing the Liver & Quieting the Spirit Acupuncture Method in the Treatment of 45 Post-stroke Insomnia Cases," *Zhong Guo Zhen Jiu (Chinese Acupuncture &*

Moxibustion), #11, 1996, p. 25

34 Chen Song-quan, "Clinical Observations on the Application of Acupuncture for Hypertension During Patients' Post-stroke Recovery Period," *Shang Hai Zhen Jiu Za Zhi (Shanghai Journal of Acupuncture & Moxibustion)*, #3, 1995, p. 109

35 One kPa = 7.5 millimeters of mercury (mmHg)

36 Zheng Zu-yan *et al.*, "Observation on the Immediate Relief of Headaches After Brain Infarction Using Bleeding Technique," *Lin Chuang Zhen Jiu (Clinical Acupuncture & Moxibustion)*, #2, 1997, p. 48

37 Tian Yuan-sheng *et al.*, "The Treatment of 80 Cases of Urinary Incontinence with Scalp Needling at *Bai Hui* (GV 20)," *Zhong Guo Zhen Jiu (Chinese Acupuncture & Moxibustion)*, #6, 1989, p. 28

38 Li Hua *et al.*, "Warm Moxibustion on *Tai Xi* (Ki 3) Point with Massage Treatment for Post-stroke Urinary Retention," *Lin Chuang Zhen Jiu Za Zhi (Journal of Clinical Acupuncture & Moxibustion)*, #3, 1997, p. 40

39 Xu Xiu-ju, "Embedding Seeds on the Auricle to Treat 62 Cases of Constipation Caused by Stroke," *Gan Su Zhong Yi (Gansu Chinese Medicine)*, #11, 2003, p. 34

40 Liu Kong-jiang, "Using Awn Needles to Treat 38 Cases of Stroke Patients with Chronic Constipation," *Zhong Guo Zhen Jiu (Chinese Acupuncture & Moxibustion)*, #12, 2003, p. 742

41 Warning: When using deep insertions of 5-6 inches, care must be taken to avoid touching the abdominal aorta and branches of the lumbar spinal nerves. The tip of the needles should be lateral to the intervertabral foramen of L3, L4, and L5.

42 Pang Hong, "Embedding Seeds on the Auricle to Treat Edema as a Result of Stroke," *Zhong Guo Zhen Jiu (Chinese Acupuncture & Moxibustion)*, #3, 1995, p. 21

43 Zhang Tong *et al.*, "The Effectiveness of Acupuncture for Post-CVA Neuralgia in Paralytic Limbs," *Zhong Yi Za Zhi (Journal of Chinese Medicine)*, #1, 2001, p. 24

44 Lu Wei-xia, The Treatment of Post-stroke Persistent Phrenospasm with Acupoint Injection Combined with Chinese Herbal Medicine for 62 Patients," *Si Chuan Zhong Yi (Sichuan Chinese Medicine)*, #2, 2003, p. 73

45 Zhang Hai-ji, "The Acupuncture Treatment for Laughing Addiction in 11 Post-stroke Cases," *Zhong Guo Zhen Jiu (Chinese Acupuncture & Moxibustion)*, #1, 1999, p. 52

SEVEN
From Art to Science

In the previous chapters, most of the emphasis has been on acupuncture's efficacy in eliminating or improving clinical signs and symptoms in post-stroke patients. In this chapter, we present abstracts of yet more clinical trials and experiments which show acupuncture's objective effects on Western medical markers in post-stroke patients and laboratory animals. These biomedical markers include serum lipids, fibrinogen, platelet cAMP, cGMP, and plasma prostaglandins as well as changes in CT scan, hemorrheological indices, and EEG tracings. In this chapter we also discuss studies which show that the combination of Western medical diagnostic procedures can help improve the selection of acupuncture protocols and increase the accuracy of prognosis of acupuncture's effects.

Human Studies

The first study concerns changes in serum HDL-C, fibrinogen, FDP, and hemorrheological indices in stroke patients due to acupuncture.[1] There were 322 patients with cerebral infarction enrolled in this study. This diagnosis was confirmed by CT scan, lumbar puncture, and EEG in 105 patients.

Seventy-six percent of the patients were between 51-70 years old. Two-thirds of them were in the first 15 days after infarction. Pertinent medical history included hypertension in 197 cases, hyperlipidemia in 81 cases, heavy smoking in 114 cases, and alcoholism in 95 cases. In terms of TCM pattern discrimination, 186 cases presented with stroke of the channels, 97 presented with stroke of the network vessels, four presented with stroke of the viscera, and 35 presented with stroke of the bowels. In addition, 63 presented with ascendant liver yang hyperactivity, 136 presented with liver-kidney yin vacuity, 67 presented with qi and blood stasis and stagnation, and 56 presented with severe phlegm and dampness.

Patients were randomly assigned to any one of four groups. Members of the acupuncture only group were needled mainly at points on the yang ming channels with auxiliary points on the tai yang and shao yang channels to free the flow of qi and blood and to balance yin and yang. Acupuncture was performed once per day on the affected side for 20 minutes per time. Twelve treatments equaled one course of treatment. In the acupuncture plus herbal medicine group, patients were administered *Bu Yang Huan Wu Tang* (Supplement Yang & Restore Five [Tenths] Decoction) to move the qi and quicken the blood in addition to the preceding acupuncture protocol. In the acupuncture plus IV drip group, an IV drip of low molecular dextran was administered daily for 15 days followed by 36 consecutive acupuncture treatments as above. The fourth group received an IV drip with a concentrated extract of *Dang Gui* (Radix Angelicae Sinensis) in glucose once per day for 15 days followed by injection of the same extract in 3-4 acupoints each time. The average number of acupoint injections in this group was 36 times.

This study showed 94% of the patients were helped by all four treatment regimens. In general, the lower limbs fared better than the upper limbs and recovery was more pronounced proximally as opposed to distally. The basically cured rate was 48.14%. This rate was 89.4% in mild cases and 3.3% in severe cases. Nonetheless, the scores in the severe cases were increased by 30.41% with treatment, a promising improvement in these patients. Both the effective rate and the cured rate also correlated positively with the duration of the disease. A cured rate of 58.08% and an effective rate of 90.01% in patients treated in the first week of their illness dropped to 34.78% and 89.86% respectively in patients one month or longer post-stroke. Forty-six patients were tested for serum lipoproteins, including cholesterol, triglycerides, beta-lipoproteins, and high density (HDL) and low density (LDL) lipoproteins. Serum HDL was markedly increased ($P < 0.01$), while beta-lipoproteins decreased ($P < 0.05$) after treatments. Blood viscosity, cholesterol, triglycerides, and fibrinogen (which were all higher than normal in these patients prior to treatment) were likewise

improved. Thirty-eight patients presented with a purple tongue indicating the presence of blood stasis, and whole blood viscosity and hematocrit in these patients were higher than those without a purple tongue. The above clinical and laboratory findings indicate that acupuncture treatment, "by regulating and promoting circulation of qi and blood," can improve the function of the affected limbs and the recovery of the patients with cerebral vascular accidents.

The second study discusses correlations of CT scan in post-stroke patients with the effectiveness of acupuncture.[2] This study consisted of 108 patients who had suffered from a CVA three weeks (67 patients) to three months (41 patients) prior to the onset of acupuncture treatment. These patients met the clinical and radiologic criteria for cerebral infarct in 79 patients and cerebral hemorrhage in 29 patients. There were 69 males and 39 females 7-84 years of age. Eighty-two patients (75.9%) were 50 years or older. Sixty-nine patients (63.9%) were classified as having severe hemiplegia, 32 had moderate hemiplegia, and seven had mild hemiplegia. All patients were mentally clear and hospitalized. CT scan of the head and skull identified the location of the lesion which showed a good correlation with their symptoms. Those that had lesions in their parietal cortex, deep foci, and multiple foci had severe paralysis. Twenty-seven of the 29 patients who had lesions located deep in the cerebrum had cerebral hemorrhage, and 41 of the aphasic patients with severe paralysis had lesions in the left cerebral hemisphere.

In addition to routine Western medical treatment, patients were treated with body acupuncture based on TCM pattern discrimination plus scalp acupuncture. Five scalp acupuncture zones were used which corresponded to the areas of dyskinesia/paresthesia of the affected extremities. Acupuncture was administered once per day for approximately one month, with one day of rest after six daily treatments. Improvement in the myodynamia of the affected limb was used as a gauge of the effectiveness of the treatment.

Of the 108 patients studied, the Chinese authors noted marked improvement in 23 patients and some improvement in an additional 67 patients. Therefore, the protocol was judged to be effective in a total of 90 patients or 83.3%. When treatment was begun within three weeks of the patient's stroke, the effective rate was raised to 90.9%. In comparison, the effective rate was only 71.4% for those who received acupuncture treatment after three weeks following onset of their illness (P < 0.05). The authors also reported on a comparison of 53 patients in the above cohort with 41 patients who were similar in terms of age and disease condition but who were treated with only routine Western medication. The total effectiveness rate in this comparison group was only 63.4%.

The study noted that the size and location of the lesions also influenced the response rate. Foci situated in the basal ganglion which were lacunar and small in area fared better than those with lesions in the internal capsules, hemisphere, brain stem, and in the temporo-occipital region which tended to be larger, deeper, and bilateral in distribution. The respective total effectiveness rates in these two groups were 78.6% versus 66%. Likewise, patients with severe paralysis associated with aphasia and/or with systemic diseases or serious complications were among the poor responders.

The next three studies all show that acupuncture can improve serum lipoproteins in post-stroke patients. The first of these studies describes the acupuncture treatment of 400 patients who had suffered cerebral thrombosis from one week up to five years prior to treatment.[3] There were 280 males and 120 females 24-76 years old with an average age of 60.4 years included in this study. Acupoints were selected along the yang ming, liver, and gallbladder channels. *Di Cang* (St 4) and *Jia Che* (St 6) were added to those with facial paralysis, and *Lian Quan* (CV 23) was added for speech problems. Thirty gauge filiform needles were used. After the qi was obtained, supplementation or drainage technique was used with needle inserted into 5-6 points. Each treatment lasted 30 minutes, and the needles were restimulated once per treatment. Twenty such treatments equaled one course of treatment series. Serum triglyceride, cholesterol, and beta-lipoprotein were compared before and after treatment.

Treatment was considered effective if the lipoprotein was lowered by 20mg % or more. Treatment was considered markedly effective if it was lowered by 50mg % or more. The study showed triglycerides were lowered by 26.9mg% in 260 patients (65%), cholesterol was lowered by 29.1mg% in 290 patients (72.5%), and beta-lipoprotein was lowered by 64.5mg% in 270 patients (67.5 %). Thus all three serum lipoproteins were significantly lowered after acupuncture therapy (P < 0.01).

The next study was a two-wing comparison trial conducted on 100 patients with CVAs of three days to three years duration.[4] All these patients also suffered from hyperlipidemia. In other words, their serum cholesterol and/or triglyceride were 10% above the upper limit of normal. The treatment group consisted of 85 patients in which 48 patients (56%) were 59 years of age or older. The duration of illness in 38 patients (44.7%) was less than 30 days. Seven of the 15 patients in the comparison group were 59 years or older. Seven patients (47%) in this group had CVAs of less than 30 days. The Western medical diagnoses of these patients included cerebral hemorrhage and thrombosis. These patients presented several different Chinese medical patterns.

In the treatment group, acupuncture was administered on the affected side using two different techniques, such as even supplementing-even draining manipulation and running needle. Bilaterally symmetrical acupuncture was also used in some cases. Three to four acupoints were used each time for 1-2 treatments per day for five days. This treatment was repeated after two days of rest. One month of treatment was considered one course of therapy.

The comparison group received vitamins, such as niacin, and *Fu Fang Dan Shen Pian* (Compound Salvia Tablets), a Chinese herbal medicine. Patients took three tablets three times per day of this medication. One month of treatment also equaled one course in this group.

This study showed that the patients treated with acupuncture had significant decreases in serum TG, LDL, and beta-lipoprotein as well as increases in HDL ($P < 0.01$). In contrast, TG continued to rise in patients in the comparison group ($P < 0.05$).When the effects of acupuncture were analyzed according to the patients' Chinese medical pattern discrimination, there were no particular patterns of changes in TC, TG, and LDL among the various patterns. However HDL increased in all patients regardless of pattern presentation. While these increases in HDL were significantly higher in females than in males treated with acupuncture,

there was no gender effect noted among other lipoproteins. The increase of HDL was also significantly higher in patients with cerebral thrombosis than those with hemorrhage. In patients with good clinical recovery, HDL and TG were improved more than the other patients. Thus the Chinese authors attributed acupuncture's benefits to stroke patients to its effect on improving their hyperlipidemia.

The following study consisted of 100 hospital inpatients with cerebral thrombosis.[5] The clinical diagnosis of these patients was confirmed by CT scan. The pertinent medical history of these patients included hypertension and atherosclerosis. The treatment group consisted of 50 patients, including 28 males and 22 females. The average age of this group was 65.5 years old, with a range of 42-79 years.

Acupuncture was performed on 7-8 points on the yang ming, liver, and gallbladder channels. Twenty-eight gauge needles were used based on the principle of supplementing vacuity and draining repletion. Each treatment lasted for 30 minutes with stimulation applied once for reinforcement. One treatment per day for 30 days equaled one course of therapy, with three days of rest between successive courses.

The comparison group also consisted of 50 patients, 26 males and 24 females. The average age of this group was 60.5 years old, with a range of 24-81 years. These patients received oral herbal medicines twice per day for seven days as one course of treatment. This treatment was repeated based on individual medical condition. The formulas used in this group were *Bu Yang Huan Wu Tang* (Supplement Yang & Restore Five [Tenths] Decoction) and *Tian Ma Gou Teng Yin* (Gastrodia & Uncaria Beverage).

Prior to treatment, baseline serum lipoproteins in these two groups of patients, both HDL and LDL, were comparable (P > 0.05). After treatment, acupuncture significantly increased the HDL and lowered the LDL (P<0.01). In contrast, only the LDL was significantly lowered in the comparison group (P < 0.05). Furthermore, the treatment group showed a more profound effect on both serum lipoproteins than the comparison group. Based on these findings, Dr. Li postulated that the technique of supplementing vacuity and draining repletion was the principle mechanism for balancing yin and yang and thereby increasing the HDL and decreasing the LDL.

Prostaglandin 12 (PGI2) is a potent vasodilator and anti-platelet factor, while thromboxane 2 (TXB2) is an effective vasoconstrictor and promotes platelet aggregation. Thus, these two factors have opposite effects on the vasculature and platelets. Each one plays an important role in maintaining the integrity of vessel walls and the homeostasis of the internal environment, the regulation of platelet function and vascular tension, and the formation of atherosclerosis, coagulation, and thrombosis. In addition, these functions are also regulated by the level of cAMP in the platelets. Therefore, the determination of the content of these substances is valuable for investigating the prevention, treatment, and mechanism of stroke with acupuncture.

The next trial studied acupuncture's effects on TXB2 and 6-Keto-PGF1a.[6] This study's cohort consisted of 63 stroke patients with upper limb paralysis. These 63 patients were equally divided into three groups. The first group received acupuncture within 1-3 days of the onset of their stroke, the second group received acupuncture 4-8 days after the occurrence of their stroke, and the third group received acupuncture 9-21 days post-stroke. Their baseline characteristics were comparable in terms of age, Fugl-Meyer motor function score, medical history, and complications. An orthogonal design study of the acupoints needled, the strength of stimulation, and the choice of alternating or combination needling of the healthy and affected side was created.

Thirty gauge needles were used at approximately 2:00 PM for 30 minutes per day. All patients also received standard Western medical treatment for cerebral infarction. Fugl-Meyer motor function scores were recorded on day two and day 45. Blood samples for plasma TXB2 and 6-keto prostaglandin F1a (6-Keto-PGF1a) were collected 24 hours after the first acupuncture treatment and on day 30.

When the preceding four parameters were analyzed, the patients 1-3 days post-stroke who received acupuncture treatment on the head and body yin and yang channels did better than the other two groups (P < 0.05). The strength of the acupuncture stimulation and the points selected for acupuncture showed no statistical difference among these three groups of patients. The plasma levels of TXB2 and 6-Keto-PGF1a corresponded directly with the observed clinical outcomes. The level of TXB2 was the lowest and 6-Keto-PGF1a was highest among patients who received acupuncture within 1-3 days post-stroke.

Based on these results, the authors concluded that patients with upper limb paralysis due to cerebral infarction are best treated in the first three days post-stroke by using acupoints on the scalp and body yin and yang channels. They further postulated that acupuncture may decrease blood vessel spasm mediated by TXB2 and thrombus formation mediated by PGF1a.

The next study evaluated the effects of acupuncture on platelet cyclic nucleotides and plasma prostaglandin in stroke patients.[7] The acupuncture treatment group consisted of 26 hospitalized patients 40-78 years old. Nineteen of these patients suffered from cerebral infarct and seven suffered from cerebral hemorrhage. All received treatment between 5-120 days post-stroke. In addition, another 12 stroke patients 51-76 years old received a variety of Western medications. These 12 patients served as the comparison group. Among them, seven had cerebral infarcts and five had cerebral hemorrhages. These patients were 7-61 days post-stroke. The Chinese medical patterns of all patients in this study were discriminated into yang hyperactivity, yin vacuity, qi vacuity, and wind and phlegm.

The treatment group received acupuncture 1-2 times per day at 3-4 acupoints. The key points were *Feng Chi* (GB 20), *Qu Chi* (LI 11), *Nei Guan* (Per 6), *San Yin Jiao* (Sp 6), and *Zu San Li* (St 36). Needling was done on the affected side with either supplementation or draining technique as appropriate. One course of treatment consisted of five consecutive daily treatments with two days of rest in between. The study period was one month for both groups. Fasting blood samples were collected before and after the completion of the study for assays of platelet cAMP, cGMP, plasma TXB2, and 6-keto-PGF1a. Plasma prostaglandin was collected on day 15.

This study showed significant increases in platelet cAMP and cGMP in the treatment group with cerebral infarction ($P < 0.01$), but no significant increase was noted in patients with cerebral hemorrhage in either the acupuncture or comparison groups. Significant increases of 6 keto-PGF1a were also seen in the treatment group after treatment ($P < 0.05$). Increased platelet cAMP

was noted only in patients presenting yin vacuity among the four traditional Chinese diagnostic patterns. In patients who were cured by acupuncture, platelet cAMP was significantly increased on day 15 and was further increased on day 30. Platelet cyclic nucleotides and plasma 6 keto-PGF1a were higher on day 15 in male patients who received acupuncture. Based on these outcomes, the authors attributed the effects of acupuncture to the increases of platelet cAMP and plasma 6-Keto-PGF1a in patients with cerebral infarction which, in turn, restored the vascular integrity and vascular tone, thus re-establishing the blood flow in the ischemic brain tissue.

The concluding human trial studied the effects of a specific acupuncture protocol on Plasma tissue plasminogen (t-PA) and plasminogen activator inhibitor (PAI-1) activities of fibrinolysis in patients with acute cerebral infarction. [8] This study consisted of 50 patients with acute cerebral thrombosis of 8-48 hours duration. Their clinical diagnoses were confirmed by CT scan. These 50 patients were divided into two groups of 25 patients each. In the treatment group, there were 16 males and nine females with a mean age of 65.48 ± 4.96 years.

These patients received *He's San Tong* acupuncture method. This included bleeding *Si Shen Cong* (M-HN-1), *Qu Ze* (Per 3), and *Wei Zhong* (Bl 54) once per day for seven days. The tongue was also bled until its color changed from dark purple to dark red. This blood-letting was followed by acupuncture at *Qu Chi* (LI 11), *Tian Shu* (St 25), *He Gu* (LI 4), *Feng Long* (St 40), *Tai Chong* (Liv 3), *Si Shen Cong* (M-HN-1), and *Zhong Wan* (CV 12). Treatment was given five times per week for three weeks. In the comparison group, there were 18 males and seven females with a mean age of 63.76 ±5.86 years. These patients received focal acupoint therapy five times per week for four weeks.

Yet another 20 patients served as a control group. This group consisted of 12 males and eight females with a mean age of 65.54 ± 6.67 years. These patients had been hospitalized for convalescence after experiencing cerebral infarctions.

(t-PA) and (PAI-1) were assayed on day two in all three groups of patients. Both tests were repeated on day seven and day 21 on the patients receiving acupuncture.

The study showed that t-PA activity was higher and PAI-1 activity was lower in the control group than in the two acupuncture groups on day two and throughout the study. On the seventh day, t-PA activity increased in both acupuncture groups when compared with their respective readings on day two (P < 0.05) and that this increase persisted through day 21. In contrast, plasma PAI-1 activity was lower in both acupuncture groups on day seven and day 21 when compared with their respective readings on day two (P < 0.05). The Chinese authors further concluded that the acute phase changes of t-PA and PAI-1 were influenced more by the *He's San Tong* method than focal point acupuncture to hasten fibrinolysis in the acute phase of cerebral infarction.

Animal Studies

Studies on animals allow for the control and quantification of the induced pathological lesions as well as the effects of the treatment. The following three studies were all conducted on rats. Cerebral ischemia was created by occlusion of the cerebral blood flow. Clinical behaviors were then correlated with pathological findings. All three of these studies showed that acupuncture improved the cerebral blood flow, lessened the volume of brain infarctions, and minimized neurological deficits. The purpose of the first study was to assess the effects of electro-acupuncture (EA) on regional cerebral blood flow (rCBF) and cerebral infarct in a rat model of acute cerebral ischemia/reperfusion.[9] Focal cortical ischemia in the middle cerebral artery distribution was achieved by arterial occlusion in both a model group (eight rats) and an EA-treated group (eight rats). A group of four rats that had sham operations were used for comparison. Occlusion of the artery was performed for one hour followed by reperfusion for one hour. Blood flow in the selected cerebral cortex was measured with laser doppler flowmeter (LDF) and recorded every five minutes. Neurological deficits were likewise evaluated on a scale of zero to seven, zero being no imbalance in activity noted and seven being inability to maintain a normal posture (thus the rat would lay on its side).

Rats were treated with electro-acupuncture at *Ren Zhong* (GV 26) and *Bai Hui* (GV 20). A 0.5 inch filiform needle was inserted vertically to one millimeter in depth. Electrical stimulus was generated using a G-6805 machine with 1.0-1.2 milliamperes intensity. Electro-acupuncture treatment lasted for 30 minutes. After the initial study, 24-hour perfusion was carried out before the rats were decapitated and the brains immediately frozen at minus 20° for 10 minutes. The brain was sectioned into two millimeter sections, fixed, and analyzed for infarction volume.

This study showed that rCBF in the middle cerebral artery distribution was significantly impaired after arterial occlusion with some improvement with reperfusion. Regional CBF in the rats in the model group decreased from 30-70% of the pre-occlusion level, with the central area of the middle cerebral artery distribution being more affected than its peripheral region. Electro-acupuncture significantly improved the CBF ($P < 0.05$). The ischemic situation was rapid in onset but transient. However, it did not return to the pre-occlusion level. When the volume of cerebral infarctions was compared, the rats that received the electro-acupuncture treatments were only one seventh of those in the model group ($P < 0.01$).

In comparing the neurological deficits of the rats studied, the deficits were higher in the model group than in the EA-treated group. The results correlated directly with the level of the rCBF impairment and the volume of cerebral infarction. The score of the EA-treated group was level one, but the model group was level seven ($P < 0.01$). Therefore, it was determined that electro-acupuncture of cerebral infarctions improved rCBF in the affected areas, decreased the areas' infarct volumes, and minimized neurological deficits in the rat models. Based on these outcomes, the authors suggested that electro-acupuncture should be started as early as possible and maintained for as long as possible.

Another experiment was conducted on Wistar rats to ascertain the effect of electro-acupuncture on cerebral ischemia.[10] Forty male rats weighing 200-250 grams each were placed into four study groups: 1) sham operation group; 2) middle cerebral artery (MCA) occlusion group, *i.e.,* the model group; 3) MCA occlusion with electro-acupuncture on single side; and 4) MCA occlusion with electro-acupuncture on both sides. Under anesthesia, MCA occlusion was achieved by inserting nylon filaments into

the MCA. Electro-acupuncture was applied to the rats in both the single-side and double-side groups. Acupoints on the left side were used for the rats in the single-side group. Both left and right sides were used on the double-side group. *He Gu* (LI 4), *Nei Guan* (Per 6), *Qu Chi* (LI 11), *Chi Ze* (Lu 5), *Zu San Li* (St 36), and *San Yin Jiao* (Sp 6) were punctured with the needles connected to Han's Electro-anesthesia Apparatus with a frequency of 3 Hertz. The intensity of the stimulus was monitored with the vibration of the animals' limbs. Electrodes were fixed to the cortex in four locations. Electroencephalogram (EEG) tracings were recorded with a RM-6000 polygraph. The changes of the frequency (times/second) and amplitude (mv of the brain waves) were monitored. Electroencephalogram recordings were obtained in the sham operation and model groups at two hours and 50 minutes. Such recordings were obtained in the single- and double-side groups at two hours and 30 minutes after the occlusion of the MCA plus another 20 minutes of electro-acupuncture. Electroencephalogram tracings were then recorded at the time the acupuncture needle was withdrawn. Electroencephalogram tracings were again recorded at 10 minute intervals for 30 seconds up to 30 minutes after the initial recording in all groups. Compar-isons of the amplitude and frequency of the EEG tracings were analyzed, and statistical differences were determined by the Student t Test.

While both the amplitude and frequency of the EEG recording were stable in the sham operation group throughout the observation period, rats in the model group had a steady but significant reduction ($P < 0.05$) in both amplitude and frequency at all the measured times. Compared with the model group, the EEG changes were significantly better in the single-side group in both the initial and all subsequent readings ($P <$

0.05). Likewise, changes were also significantly better (P < 0.05) for the double-side group than the single-side group up to the 20-minute recordings. Both the amplitude and frequency of the EEG tracings were not significantly different among the three groups with MCA occlusion at the 30-minute recording. This experiment provides EEG evidence suggesting that electro-acupuncture can improve cerebral function in those with cerebral ischemia.

The following experiment evaluated the effect of electro-acupuncture on the cerebral function in male Wistar rats after transient middle cerebral artery occlusion (MCAO).[11] Twelve-week old, male rats with a body weight of 250-280 grams were divided into two groups—a treatment group which received electro-acupuncture and a comparison group which received no treatment. The treatment group was further subdivided into two groups depending on the different acupoints chosen. Group A received treatment at *Ren Zhong* (GV 26) and *Bai Hui* (GV 20), while group B was treated at *Han Yan* (GB 4), *Xuan Lu* (GB 5), *Xuan Li* (GB 6), and *Qu Bin* (GB 7). Each experiment consisted of 13 rats per group with body temperatures maintained at 37° C under anesthesia. Middle cerebral artery occlusion was achieved using nylon fiber for 90 minutes. The rats were then returned to their cages. Animal behavior, including cerebral nutrition, walking, and balancing, were recorded by independent observers according to the Zea Longa assessment method at 24 hours after MCAO and every six days thereafter up until day 30. Electro-acupuncture was performed on the two treatment subgroups. Under anesthesia, 0.35mm x 40mm needles were inserted 0.3-0.5 inches into the acupoints. The needles were connected to an Olim Pulse LFP 4000A Apparatus using a three mA current with a frequency of 3/20Hz.

Electro-acupuncture was conducted for 30 minutes every other day for 30 days. On the 30th day, the animals were decapitated and their brains were sectioned in two millimeter thick sections and stained with a 2% TCC solution followed by formalin fixation. The infarct area was photographed by a digital camera (Sony DSC-P71) and calculated using ADOBE Photoshop v5.0. The volume of infarct was the product of the infarcted area times two millimeters in thickness. This experiment was repeated five times. Behavior assessments were tallied and analyzed using the Student t Test. Brain infarct volume was analyzed by ANOVA.

At day six, assessment of behavior showed better recovery in the two electro-acupuncture subgroups than the no-treatment group. In terms of comparison between the two subgroups which received electro-acupuncture, the rats in group B were statistically better in balancing and walking at day 24. It was also noted that the survival rate was higher in group B rats. The volume of brain infarct was largest in the no-treatment group. The brain infarct volume was likewise smaller in group B than in group A. Based on these findings, the Chinese authors concluded that electro-acupuncture can improve motor, sensory, and intellectual functions in rats after a transient MCAO. The beneficial effect was attributed to its ability to repair the ischemic damage to the brain tissue. The authors also postulated that the electro-acupuncture may promote the recovery of cerebral function.

The Combination of Human & Animal Studies

Most current Chinese research on stroke has focused on the treatment of the sequelae of stroke as a result of untimely and improper emergency measures. The study reported on below describes bleeding the 12 hand well points as an emergency treatment in stroke patients.[12] The authors then go on to attempt to elucidate the mechanism of how the treatment works in animals. In this study, there were 55 patients with deranged speech who had just experienced a stroke. These 55 patients were divided into two groups—a treatment group and a comparison group. Thirty-three patients were in the treatment group and 22 patients were in the comparison group. Based on their clinical presentation, the patients were further subdivided into mild, moderate, and severe categories. Patients in both groups were monitored for blood pressure, respiration, heart rate, and level of consciousness. The treatment group received blood-letting at the 12 hand well points. Following treatment patients in the treatment group had increased heart rate and improved consciousness. The systolic blood pressure also increased in the mild cases. Rheology was measured in 29 patients using 3D-TCD apparatus prior to administered the bleeding therapy. It was noted that the blood flow in the main cerebral arteries was variable—either fast or slow. Bleeding of the 12 hand well points regulated this abnormal blood flow towards normal.

To explain the mechanisms behind these outcomes, acute cerebral ischemia was induced by legation of the common carotid artery in rabbits. Bleeding of the 12 hand well points in these rabbits improved the low amplitude of the rheo-encephalograph (REG) induced by acute ischemia. This effect, which was sustained for a long time, was better than that from the administration of nicotinic acid and its derivatives. In an experiment inducing cerebral hematoma in rabbits, the amplitude of the brain waves shown in REG also improved due to bleeding the six hand well

points. Even better results were obtained if this technique was performed on the affected side. However, when a more simplified bleeding of three hand well points was employed, it was less effective. Bleeding of three hand well points on the yin channels showed no effect at all. These results agreed with the principle that "The yang channels go to the head, [and] the yin channels do not." From these outcomes, the authors concluded that the positive effects of bleeding the 12 hand well points in acute cerebral ischemia is due to a combination of bleeding, pain, and the acupoints.

In yet another experiment on rabbits in which the radial, ulnar, and median nerves of the paw were severed bilaterally, the effects of the bleeding of the 12 hand well points were found to still be effective although weakened. However, when Lidocaine was applied to block the sympathetic nerves on the wall of the brachial arteries and veins, the treatment was completely ineffective. This observation suggested that somatic and sympathetic nerves on the blood vessel walls are the major pathways for the treatment to affect the REG. To clarify how the mechanism of this treatment worked, blocking agents such as atropine, phentolamine, and propanolol were injected into the rabbit's cerebral ventricles followed by bleeding the 12 hand well points. This showed that the changes in REG occurred through the regulation of the cholinergic and adrenergic nerves. The alpha and M-receptors also played an important role.

When cerebral ischemia occurred in a cohort of large rats, nerve excitability increased. As a result, excitatory amino acids (EAA) increased which led to the opening of the calcium channels on the cell membrane. This resulted in increased intracellular calcium and heightened the activity of CaM leading to a series of pathological reactions and brain cell death. In another experiment with rats, the middle cerebral artery was ligated leading to cerebral ischemia causing a significantly decreased intracellular calcium concentration in the affected area. Within three minutes of cerebral ischemia, the 12 well points were bled. After bleeding, the extracellular calcium concentration was significantly less than that of the rats who were not treated. This observation suggested that the bleeding technique might play an important role in preventing the calcium influx into the brain cells and minimize cell injury and death. In the same brain ischemic model, anaerobic glycolysis also increased in the affected area. Treatment with bleeding the 12 hand well points lowered the hydrogen in the ischemic brain tissue. Likewise, the treatment described above maintained membrane stability better and reduced intracellular edema by significantly reducing the leaking of intracellular potassium and extracellular sodium in the ischemic brain cells.

Endnotes

[1] Oi L.Y. et al., "Observation on Acupuncture Treatment of 322 Cases of Cerebral Infarction and Changes in Serum HDL-C, Fibrinogen, FDP, Hemorrheological Indices, Etc. During Treatment," *International Journal of Clinical Acupuncture*, #1, 1990, p. 39-46

[2] Fang Yuan et al., "CT Scanning & the Therapeutic Effects of Acupuncture on 108 Cases of Hemiplegia Due to Apoplexy," *International Journal of Clinical Acupuncture*, #1, 1990, p. 1-6

[3] Xu Yu-min, "Observations on Acupuncture Compared to Changes in Serum Lipids in Those with Ischemic Stroke," *Shang Hai Zhen Jiu Za Zhi (Shanghai Journal of Acupuncture & Moxibustion)*, #2, 1992, p. 13

[4] Li Zong-ren et al., "Clinical Observations on the Effects of Acupuncture on Hyperlipidemia in Stroke Patients," *Zhong Guo Zhen Jiu (Chinese Acupuncture & Moxibustion)*, #4, 1988, p. 28-32

[5] Li Yang, "The Effects of Acupuncture on Serum Lipoproteins in Patients with Cerebral Thrombosis," *Zhong Guo Zhen Jiu (Chinese Acupuncture & Moxibustion)*, #7, 1996, p. 7-8

[6] Li Yang, "The Selection of the Optimum Acupuncture Treatment Program for Paralysis of the Upper Limb Due to Cerebral Infarction and Its Effects on the Content of TXB2 & 6-Keto-PGF1a," *Zhong Guo Zhen Jiu (Chinese Acupuncture & Moxibustion)*, #7, 1996, p. 7-8

[7] Li Zhong-ren et al., "The Influence of Acupuncture on Blood Platelet cAMP, cGMP, Plasma PGI2, and TXB2 Contents in Apoplectic Patients," *International Journal of Clinical Acupuncture*, #2, 1990, p. 113-117

[8] Wang Lin-peng et al., "The Effects of He's San Tong Acupuncture on Plasma t-PA & PAI-1 Activities of Fibrinolysis in Patients with Acute Cerebral Infarction," *Zhong Guo Zhen Jiu (Chinese Acupuncture & Moxibustion)*, #11, 2003, p. 681-683

[9] Zhou Fei et al., "The Effect of Electro-acupuncture on Cerebral Infarction & Neurological Deficits Correlated with Regional Cerebral Flow & Infarction Volume in Rat Models with Acute Focal Cerebral Ischemia," *Shang Hai Zhen Jiu Za Zhi (Shanghai Journal of Acupuncture & Moxibustion)*, #5, 2003, p. 3-6

[10] Jia Qing-shun et al., "The Influence of Different Electro-acupuncture Modes on EEG in Local Cerebral Ischemia in Rats," *International Journal of Clinical Acupuncture*, #4, 2002, p. 283-287

[11] Wang Shao-jun et al., "The Beneficial Effects of Electro-acupuncture on Cerebral Functions in Rats with Middle Cerebral Artery Occlusion," *Liao Ning Zhong Yi Za Zhi (Liaoning Journal of Chinese Medicine)*, #9, 2003, p. 750-751

[12] Guo Yi et al., "Clinical & Laboratory Studies on Bleeding the Hand 12 Well Points," *Shang Hai Zhen Jiu Za Zhi (Shanghai Journal of Acupuncture & Moxibustion)*, #2, 1997, p. 11-12

EIGHT
Prevention

According to the first chapter of the *Nei Jing: Su Wen (Inner Classic: Simple Questions)*, treating disease after it has occurred is like beginning to dig a well after one has already become thirsty, whereas the prevention of disease in a seemingly healthy person is the hallmark of the superior physician. This suggests that Chinese medicine has a long history of promoting the importance of preventive care. The prevention of stroke is especially important because dealing with the consequences of stroke involves long-term care and is a great deal more costly and painful. By understanding the risk factors and noticing the warning signs, a person can determine whether one needs the timely use of professional therapies to prevent a cerebrovascular accident (CVA or stroke). Beginning with diet, exercise, sleep habits, prescription drugs, Chinese medicine, and other therapies, stroke (whether an ischemic or hemorrhagic CVA) can best be prevented using a multidimensional approach.

A stroke occurs when an artery to the brain becomes clogged by a blood clot (ischemic stroke) or when an artery to the brain bursts (hemorrhagic stroke). This cuts off the blood and oxygen supply to a part of the brain. Brain cells lose function within minutes of oxygen deprivation. As a result, the part of the body controlled by the oxygen-deprived brain cells cannot function. Using the risk factor information below, patients and practitioners can calculate their or their patients' chances of having a stroke. This calculation will determine the amount of attention that is needed to prevent a stroke. In other words, we can take charge of reducing or eliminating many risk factors.

Risk Factors That Can Be Changed

Hypertension

High blood pressure or hypertension is the single greatest risk factor for stroke. It is estimated to play a role in about 70% of all ischemic and hemorrhagic strokes. This risk is approximately four times greater if blood pressure is 160/95mmHg or above compared to those with pressures of 140/90mmHg or below. Hypertension is believed to accelerate atherogenesis (the formation of masses of plaque within the walls of degenerated, thickened arteries). Obesity, family history, diabetes, inactivity, and excess dietary sodium and alcohol intake are risk factors for the development of hypertension. People with diastolic blood pressure measurements of 90-95mmHg or higher and with systolic pressures higher then 160mmHg should receive antihypertensive therapy.[1] A study of 519 patients determined that 67% of people with morning blood pressure surges of 55mmHg or greater suffered multiple strokes compared to 33% of patients with lower morning blood pressure increases.[2] Despite widespread use of antihypertensive medications, appropriate control of hypertension is achieved in only approximately 31% of the population.[3] With lifestyle changes, alternative therapies, and drugs, more can and should be done to lower blood pressures to prevent the reduced quality of life that comes with stroke.

Atherosclerosis, Lipid Levels & Beyond

People at risk for stroke are similar to people at risk for heart attack due to their unstable atherosclerotic plaques. The current state of the arteries is seen with an intima media thickness (IMT) scan. The IMT scan shows the size and location of actual cholesterol plaque, whether or not the plaque is soft (dangerous) or hard (calcified, *i.e.*, less dangerous) as well as the thickness or "age" of the wall of the artery, thus indicating the extent of one's atherosclerosis. Cardio Risk Ultrasound, Inc. has FDA-approved software and excellent quality control with scanning of the inner two layers of the arteries. They can be reached at *www.CardioRisk.US* or 1-888-724-7484.

Testing for markers in addition to the basic cholesterol test is indicated if one is found to have atherosclerosis. High levels of total cholesterol (TC) and low-density lipoprotein (LDL, so-called bad cholesterol), elevated triglycerides (TC), and low levels of high-density lipoprotein (HDL, so-called good cholesterol) contribute to stroke. Although risk can be determined by these standard cholesterol tests, it is much more accurate to use the new generation of screening tests such as small LDL, Apo B, HDL2B, high-sensitivity C-reactive protein (CRP), fibrinogen, Chlamydia pneumoniae, insulin, homocysteine, Lp(a), and Apo E. One study has shown that high homocysteine levels led to a three-time increase in the likelihood of stroke among young women—the same as smoking a pack of cigarettes a day.[4] Elevated levels of lipoprotein a [Lp(a)] increase one's risk for coronary artery disease by 300%, even if everything else is normal.[5] Studies have found that each of these markers can be influenced by lifestyle, diet, supplements, and/or medication. Further IMT scanning can then be used to monitor improvements in atherosclerotic burden. Showing documentation about the blood tests to one's doctor may be helpful, since busy practitioners often find it difficult to keep up with the amounts of new science reported daily. The documentation in research cardiologist Dr. Superko's book, *Before the Heart Attacks*, should be adequate.

Contraceptives & hormone replacement therapy (HRT)

The low-dose oral contraceptives (OCs) used today are still associated with a risk of stroke. In a randomized, controlled study with over 10,000 women called the Women's Health Initiative, researchers found that postmenopausal women taking estrogen with or without progestin had a greater risk of stroke compared to those taking a placebo.[6]

Cigarette smoking

A recent meta-analysis found that smokers have a 50% higher risk of stroke than non-smokers. There is definite evidence that smoking itself has a direct causal effect on stroke.[7] Smoking has been shown to cause 3.7 times more hemorrhagic strokes.[8] Women who smoke and use HRT or OCs have an even higher risk of blood clots. This may be due to increased oxidative stress from smoking contributing to (blood vessel) endothelial dysfunction.[9]

Diabetes

People with diabetes have a higher risk of ischemic stroke than the general population. Evidence is growing that controlling blood sugar may lower stroke risk. Uncontrolled diabetes is linked with an increased risk of stroke. Carotid artery IMT has been shown to be greater in non-insulin-dependent diabetes mellitus (NIDDM) patients than in control subjects. In the study that uncovered this link, the main determinants of IMT in NIDDM patients were related to both post-glucose insulin levels and abnormal lipoprotein profiles characteristic of NIDDM and insulin resistance syndrome. Based on this research, it is postulated that treatment of insulin and lipoprotein levels is likely to reduce the atherosclerotic burden in NIDDM patients.[10]

Carotid stenosis

Patients who have a carotid artery (in the neck, supplying blood to the brain) that is narrowed by build-up of atherosclerotic plaque have a threefold greater risk of stroke than the general population.[11] At every level of risk factor exposure, there is substantial variation of atherosclerosis.[12]

Intima media thickness scanning is a meas-urement of subclinical disease that is useful for improving stroke prediction. B-mode ultrasound looks at the structural make-up of the inner two layers of the carotid artery. Studies have shown that echolucent carotid plaques with low integrated back-scatter (IBS) values predicted coronary plaque complexity and the development of future coronary complications in patients with stable coronary artery disease (CAD).[13]

As mentioned above, CardioRisk has FDA-approved software with well-trained ultrasound clinicians and the strictest quality control. This noninvasive carotid ultrasound can measure the current state of the disease. With equipment measuring to 0.003 millimeters, it can determine from year to year if lifestyle and other changes have improved one's atherosclerotic burden or if other treatments are necessary to prevent stroke.

Atrial fibrillation (AF)

Atrial fibrillation causes 75,000 strokes per year. This hidden cause of stroke needs to be treated first by preventing blood clots, then by restoring normal heart rate and heart rhythm. Treating "average" AF patients (*i.e.*, those with a 5% per year risk of stroke) with the anticlotting drug warfarin prevents about 30 strokes per thousand while it causes at least two episodes of major hemorrhage each year. Treating AF patients with aspirin has been shown to prevent about 15 strokes per thousand each year.[14]

Alcohol abuse

Habitual alcohol intake in excess of two drinks almost doubles the risk of stroke. More than moderate alcohol consumption significantly raises the risk of hemorrhagic stroke. The American Heart Association (AHA) does not recommend the drinking of any alcohol, as drinking pure grape juice can attain any of the benefits of wine's bioflavenoids. The AHA defines moderate drinking to two drinks for men and one drink for women per day. In a meta-analysis published in the *Journal of the American Medical Association (JAMA)*, it was found that more than five glasses of alcohol per day increased the overall risk of stroke by 64%. Heavy drinking increased the risk of ischemic stroke by 69%, compared with those who abstained.[15]

Stimulant use

Stimulants, such as cocaine and amphetamines, can cause cerebral hemorrhage as well as heart rhythm abnormalities and heart attack. Over-the-counter (OTC) drugs containing phenylpropalolamine (PPA) have definitively been linked with hemorrhagic stroke and have been taken off the market. Researchers are looking into similar risks associated with other drugs like ephedra. COX-2 inhibitors may need to be avoided if there is a stroke risk because they have a potential for accentuating bleeding and raising blood pressure.[16]

Sedentary lifestyle

People who are physically inactive are almost three times as likely to suffer a stroke than people who exercise regularly.[17]

Obesity

Obesity increases the risk of stroke by 50-100%. A waist circumference of greater than 40 inches in men and 35 inches in women is a good predictor of ischemic stroke.[18] According to Superko and Tucker:

> The danger in fat deposited around the waist is that this fat is more insulin resistant than

the kind that's stored under the skin. So the body has to keep calling for more and more insulin to deal with the fat that's stored in the belly and that means that there's more atherogenic insulin in the blood-stream if you're heavy around the waist.[19]

Hemochromatosis

Hemochromatosis is a disease of iron overload in the body. Iron overload increases clotting. Left untreated, this can lead to stroke.[20]

Dehydration or sinus infections

Dehydration or sinus infections inhibit blood flow from the brain. Venous stroke is caused by a blood clot blocking the veins that drain blood out of the brain. Therefore, dehydration and sinus infections have been linked with stroke risk.[21]

C-reactive protein (CRP)

People with blood levels of CRP above three milligrams per liter (3mg/L) are at increased risk for ischemic stroke as well as for heart attack.[22] A CRP test measures inflammation in the body. High CRP levels can point to any of the following treatable conditions: atherosclerosis, bacterial or viral infection, diabetes, gingivitis, periodontal disease, high blood pressure, inflammation of the arteries, metabolic syndrome, obesity, rheumatoid arthritis, and smoking.

Risk Factors That Cannot Be Changed

According to the authors of *HopkinsWhite Papers.com*, the following risk factors for stroke cannot be changed.[23] The presence of these risk factors should alert people to their greater srtoke risk and to the need to reduce the previously-cited risk factors that they can change.

Age

Seventy-two percent of people who suffer from stroke are older than 65 years of age.[24]

Gender

The risk of stroke is less in pre-menopausal women due to the protective effect of estrogen.

Family history

Stroke risk is greater in people whose parents or siblings have had a stroke.

Race

Blacks, Asian-Pacific Islanders, and Hispanics have a greater risk of death and disability from stroke than do whites.[25] The death rate from stroke in African Americans is almost double that of Caucasians. According to Ruland:

> Our data indicate poor rates of awareness, treatment, and control of diabetes, hypertension, and high cholesterol among study participants—African-Americans with previous stroke at the time of study enrollment... Physician attitudes, problems with patient access to care, unawareness of the importance of routine screening, and compliance with treatment are several possible reasons for the increased death rate.[26]

Prior history of stroke

About 13% of prior stroke patients have another stroke within a year, and the risk of stroke in each successive year after that is 6%.[27]

Transient ischemic attacks (TIAs)

About 36% of people who have had one or more TIAs will eventually have a full-blown stroke.[28]

Obstructive sleep apnea (OSA)

Carotid artery walls are thicker in patients with severe sleep apnea syndrome. Strong evidence exists that this increase in thickness is a valid marker of the risk of stroke. Patients with OSA are likely at risk of stroke regardless of whether or not they have other risk factors.[29] Acupuncture may help sleep apnea.

Accidents & other circumstances

Bone fractures, open heart surgery, pneumothorax, or too rapid an ascent from deep waters can result in blood clots that can lead to cerebral embolism. Head injury can cause a hemorrhagic stroke. Mild kidney dysfunction also may raise the risk of stroke.[30] Mild kidney dysfunction may be improved with Chinese herbs according to Chinese medical texts and a number of Chinese medical practitioners.

When Should Something Be Done?

This depends on the category of symptoms.

In healthy and young patients

No care is needed except to maintain a healthy way of eating and regular exercise of a half hour at least three times per week.

In those experiencing some change in how they feel

Self-care is advised. Most elderly have some change in hemodynamic viscosity of the blood (see Chapter 7). Though patients may not be receiving consistent medical care at this time, their hemodynamic index can place them in the symptomatic category below.

In those experiencing some changes in how they feel and some stroke symptoms

The initial stage of cerebral arteriosclerosis (the precursor to ischemic strokes) may present with some neurological dysfunction but is usually asymptomatic. Several techniques exist to identify potential problems before they become major ones. Therefore, one should test for arteriosclerosis, high blood pressure, or inflammation and inquire about risky eating or behavioral habits. A stroke may happen suddenly, but it often follows years of a slow build-up of fatty deposits inside the blood vessels.

Nevertheless, there do exist "hidden" warning signs easily detected by funduscopy of the retinal arterioles, by a stethoscope listening to the neck arteries, or ultrasound of the neck arteries. Intense self-care in addition to professional care is advised at this stage.

In symptomatic persons

If one experiences symptoms such as dropping utensils when eating, they should not wait for a clear Western medical diagnosis before beginning professional remedial treatment. As authors of this book, we suggest the patient be treated with Chinese medicine. Transient ischemic attacks often show nothing on tests or the diagnosis may be Parkinson's disease. About 10% of strokes are preceded by TIAs, and full-blown strokes occur in one-third of patients who have had a TIA. Therefore, even though the symptoms resolve within 24 hours, it is still very important to seek prompt help for a TIA. These are excellent opportunities to prevent permanent damage, as the risk of ischemic stroke is highest soon after a TIA. Multi-infarct dementia is caused by a series of minor strokes, and patients' abilities decline in a step-like pattern.

In those where TIA frequency has increased

If the frequency of TIAs has increased, one should not wait longer than a few hours to begin some sort of preventive treatment. Prompt medical attention by a neurologist or surgeon can prevent a fatal or disabling stroke from occurring. Brain damage may be arrested or reversed with thrombolytics or "clot-busters." These include anticoagulants that may prevent further stroke if used within three hours as well as long-term blood-thinners.

Symptoms of Emergency

1. Sudden weakness, numbness, or paralysis of the face, arm, or leg
2. Loss of speech or trouble talking or understanding speech
3. Dimness or loss of vision, particularly if only in one eye
4. Unexplained dizziness, unsteadiness, or sudden falls
5. Sudden, severe headache
6. Disorientation, confusion, or memory loss
7. Balance or coordination problems that may fluctuate over a few days

Treatments with clot-busting drugs provided within three hours of symptoms may help prevent brain damage. Hence it is extremely important to call 911 immediately if any of these symptoms of stroke occur.

Additional Warning Signs of an Impending Stroke [31]

Dizziness

In Chinese medicine, dizziness is considered a huge risk factor for stroke resulting from ascendant liver yang hyperactivity or liver wind stirring internally. Liver-kidney yin vacuity, kidney qi vacuity, or emptiness of the sea of marrow can also cause dizziness.

Index finger numbness

In Chinese medicine, numbness in an index finger indicates damp phlegm is lodged in or blocking the channels or vessels. This is considered a risk factor of great concern.

Western diagnosis of carpal tunnel syndrome (CTS)

Qi and blood stasis and stagnation of the forearm may be a signal for stroke if the mechanism of injury causing CTS is not clear or present.

Blood tests

Either high or low erythrocyte count can trigger stroke. Clinically, an elevated hematocrit typically manifests as reddening of the skin or erythema. A low hematocrit indicates anemia and points to danger of an anemia infarct.

Steps for Preventing a Stroke

Take precautions

Most people who see the above risk factors and yet take no precautions, go on to have a stroke. Besides addressing the risk factors we can change, below are additional precautions one should take whenever risk factors for impending stroke become apparent.[32]

Avoid exhaustion

Exhaustion may trigger a stroke according to Chinese medical theory because it damages the spleen. Because the spleen governs the movement and transformation of water and fluids, and phlegm is nothing other than congealed dampness, spleen vacuity commonly results in an increase in phlegm. Because blood and fluids flow together, phlegm easily causes blood stasis by blocking the free flow of the qi and blood.

Avoid outbursts of anger

In Chinese medicine, anger is the affect of the liver. Anger, especially rage, damages the liver and leads to internal stirring of liver wind that rises up to harass the head and its orifices. Even according to modern Western medicine, type A blood types characteristically have more sudden anger and have an increased risk of stroke.

Avoid worrying

Thought is the affect of the spleen, and worry is an excess of thought. Therefore, worrying damages the spleen, resulting in phlegm which eventually also causes blood stasis.

Avoid wallowing in sadness

Sadness is the affect of the lungs, and the lungs control the qi of the whole body. Therefore, excessive sadness damages the lungs, eventually damaging other organs as well. In particular, the heart and lung qi have a close relationship. Both make up the chest qi. If the lung qi becomes vacuous and insufficient due to excessive sadness, so typically will the heart qi. Then the heart will not move the blood, the blood will become static, and the channels and vessels may be struck with stroke. Further, the lungs and liver have a reciprocal, interdependent relationship in terms of the free flow of the qi. If the lung qi becomes vacuous and weak, the lungs will fail to control the liver which may become depressed or more depressed. If liver depression transforms into heat, this heat may cause yang hyperactivity or stirring of internal liver wind.

Avoid increasing fear

According to Chinese medical theory, fear damages the kidneys and the heart. In this case, kidney water may not nourish the liver and kidney yang may not help in the engenderment of heart qi. A malnourished liver may result in liver depression qi stagnation which may further evolve into blood stasis, phlegm dampness, ascendant liver yang hyperactivity, and/or internal stirring of liver wind. If kidney yang does not contribute to the warming and steaming of the heart qi, this may also lead to blood stasis and blood stasis may lead to phlegm engenderment.

Avoid constipation

The large intestine receives the turbid fraction of the by-products of digestion and re-absorbs water from these wastes. The remainder of these wastes are excreted as feces. If the turbid is not eliminated on a timely basis with a daily bowel movement, various accumulations will develop, such as heat and blood stasis but also even phlegm. In Chinese medicine, constipation is associated with a wide variety of patterns of disharmony and should be treated promptly.

Avoid rich, fatty foods

Rich, fatty foods damage the spleen. Because the spleen is the root of the engenderment and transformation of qi and blood, spleen vacuity due to rich, fatty foods may give rise to blood vacuity failing to nourish the liver. Because the spleen governs the movement and transformation of water fluids, it may also give rise to the engenderment of phlegm dampness. If this phlegm and dampness hinder and obstruct the free flow of the yang qi, this may transform depressive heat giving rise to a combination of phlegm heat. This phlegm may then

block the channels and vessels and this heat may engender wind.

Avoid alcohol

In Chinese medicine, alcohol is seen as being both hot and damp. Its dampness damages the spleen and its heat consumes yin and damages the liver. As we have seen, damage to either the spleen or liver can set in motion disease mechanisms that lead to stroke.

Avoid overeating in general

Overeating damages the spleen and stomach by inhibiting the qi mechanism. This may lead to or aggravate liver depression qi stagnation which may then lead to liver heat and yang hyperactivity. Overeating may also lead to spleen vacuity with the ultimate engenderment of blood stasis and phlegm blocking and obstructing the channels and vessels.

Be moderate in sex

Sex may likewise be a trigger for stroke. This is because excess sex, called bedroom taxation in Chinese, depletes kidney essence and may contribute to kidney yin not watering or nourishing the liver. This then leads to the engenderment of internal liver wind from hyperactivity of liver yang.

Preventing Stroke With Professionally Prescribed Chinese Medicine

Within Chinese medicine as a whole, there are the specialties of herbal medicine, acupuncture-moxibustion, tuina, and qigong. In the U.S. and China, many practitioners employ a combination of some or all these modalities to help their patients. Internally administered Chinese herbal formulas should be based on each patient's professionally diagnosed patterns or needs. Because different patients with the same disease present different patterns, a single formula designed to treat a specific pattern will not fit every patient. Nevertheless, we can identify the commonly used Chinese medicinals for the prevention and treatment of stroke. These include:

He Shou Wu (Radix Polygoni Multiflori)
Shan Zha (Fructus Crataegi)
Ze Xie (Rhizoma Alismatis)
Shi Jue Ming (Concha Haliotidis)
San Qi (Radix Notoginseng)
Huang Jing (Rhizoma Polygonati)
Hu Zhang (Rhizoma Polygoni Cuspidati)
Di Long (Pheretima)
Gou Teng (Ramulus Uncariae Cum Uncis)
Dan Shen (Radix Salviae Miltiorrhizae)
Yin Chen Hao (Herba Artemisiae Scopariae)

All of these herbal medicinals are known to decrease triglycerides in the blood. However, because *He Shou Wu* supplements the blood, it should not be used in those with a higher than normal hematocrit.

Commonly used formulas in clinical practice[33]

The following formulas are given as an idea of the kinds of formulas a professional practitioner might prescribe a patient for the prevention of stroke. Typically, these formulas would only be used as a guide or base, and additions to and subtractions from them would be made in order to tailor the medicinal ingredients to each individual's personally presenting patterns, signs and symptoms.

For **qi vacuity**, *Bu Zhong Yi Qi Tang* (Supplement the Center & Boost the Qi Decoction) is commonly used.

For **blood vacuity**, one can use *Si Wu Tang* (Four Materials Decoction) as the base formula.

For **phlegm obstruction**, *Wen Dan Tang* (Warm the Gallbladder Decoction) is commonly used as the base.

For **yin vacuity**, *Liu Wei Di Huang Wan* (Six Flavors Rehmannia Pills) are the standard formula.

For **yang vacuity**, *You Gui Wan* (Restore the Right [Kidney] Pills) are commonly the choice.

For **ascendant liver yang hyperactivity**, one can add *Long Dan Cao* (Radix Gentianae), *Sheng Di* (uncooked Radix Rehmanniae), and *Ju Hua* (Flos Chrysanthemi Morifolii) to many different formulas.

For **TIAs**, one might consider *Er Ma Si Feng Tang* (Two Ma's & Four Winds Decoction). Transient ischemic attacks often present as a pattern of yin vacuity with yang hyperactivity and stirring of wind for which this formula is indicated. It consists of:

Tian Ma (Rhizoma Gastrodiae), 10g
Luo Bu Ma (Folium Apocyni Veneti), 30g
Niu Xi (Radix Achyranthis Bidentatae), 15g
Di Long (Pheretima), 15g
Xia Ku Cao (Spica Prunellae), 15g
Hai Zao (Sargassum), 20g
Gou Teng (Ramulus Uncariae Cum Uncis), 20g
Ju Hua (Folium Chrysanthemi Morifolii), 15g

Huai Hua Zi (Flos Immaturus Sophorae
   Japonicae), 15g
Du Zhong (Cortex Eucommiae), 15g
Sang Ji Sheng (Herba Taxilli), 15g
Yi Mu Cao (Herba Leonuri), 30g

After taking the above *Er Ma Si Feng Tang*,
the patient should feel better and show
fewer symptoms of yang hyperactivity and
internal wind. Then change the formula to
Qi Ju Di Huang Wan (Lycium & Chrysan-
themum Rehmannia Pills) for 1-2 months.
This is a good formula to supplement the
kidneys and liver, enrich yin and nourish
the blood. Typically, patients can take this
ready-made medicine for long periods of
time.

If phlegm and blood stasis are pronounced,
with symptoms like dizziness, headache,
chest oppression, decreased appetite, a purple facial complexion and lips, a dark, red,
enlarged tongue, enlarged veins, and a
forceful, bowstring pulse, one might prescribe *Di Tan Huo Xue Tang* (Wash Away
Phlegm & Quicken the Blood Decoction):

Gua Lou Shi (Fructus Trichosanthis), 15-
   30g
Dan Nan Xing (bile-processed Rhizoma
   Arisaematis), 5-10g
Ban Xia (Rhizoma Pinelliae), 10g
Bai Zhu (Rhizoma Atractylodis
   Macrocephalae), 12g
Chen Pi (Pericarpium Citri Reticulatae),
   10g
Dan Shen (Radix Salviae Miltiorrhizae),
   30g
Tian Ma (Rhizoma Gastrodiae), 10g
Zhi Shi (Fructus Immaturus Aurantii), 10g

When the patient feels better, switch to *Si
Jun Zi Wan* (Four Gentlemen Pills) com-
bined with *Yi Guan Jian* (One Link
Decoction).

Other Chinese Medical Self-care Methods to Help Reduce Stroke Risk[34]

Combing & tapping on the head

Because strokes occur in the head, using the
fingers like a comb to comb the head can
help increase circulation to the brain and
thus help prevent stroke. Then tap from *Bai
Hui* (GV 20) to *Nao Hu* (GV 17) and then
also to *Shen Ting* (GV 24). Next, use the
two hands to tap gently along the bladder
and gallbladder channels for 2-3 minutes.
However, this technique is contraindicated
if the patient has high blood pressure.

Massaging the palms

Massage the center of the palms around the
acupoint *Lao Gong* (Per 8) until the palms
turn warm. Then use acupressure on *Nei
Guan* (Per 6) and *Chi Ze* (Lu 5).

Rub & cup the hands

Rub the hands together as fast as possible
until they turn very warm and then use the
palms of the hands to cup the eyes or ears
depending on the individual's need for
improving vision or hearing.

Massaging the soles, feet & legs

Use the fist on *Yong Quan* (Ki 1). Also
massage *Zhao Hai* (Ki 6), *Tai Chong* (Liv
3), and *San Yin Jiao* (Sp 6).

Self-moxibustion

Use indirect moxa on *Zu San Li* (St 36).
Moxa on *Xuan Zhong* (GB 39) is a special
method for treating high blood pressure.
Other texts specify only self-moxibustion
on *Tai Chong* (Liv 3) and *San Yin Jiao*
(Sp 6).

Train & increase the use of the nondominant hand

Since 60% of strokes happen on the right side of the brain, there is a belief that using one's left hand in daily life will result in stimulating the right side of the brain more. This stimulation may prevent some strokes.

Acupressure

The following acupressure protocol should be done under the supervision of a professional. Acupressure after an extended series of acupuncture treatments can prolong the acupuncture's therapeutic effects. Doing this protocol one half hour before going to bed helps promote deep sleep. The points include those on the nape of the neck, the temple, the vertex, around the eyes, around the ears, around the temporomandibular joint (TMJ), and especially the extra-channel point *Nei Ru* located between *Si Zhu Kong* (TB 23) and *Tong Zi Liao* (GB 1).[35]

Qigong

Qigong means literally energy work. There are a number of different forms of such energy work. However, the two main forms are moving and still qigong. Still qigong is essentially a form of meditation. It has been found at the Shanghai High Blood Pressure Research Center that quiet sitting qigong for 20-30 minutes per day reduces both blood pressure and heart rate. Further testing demonstrated this type of meditation had better results than taking high blood pressure medication.

Acupuncture & moxibustion[36]

Acupuncturists can teach patients to do simple self-care moxibustion treatments as mentioned above. However, high stroke risk patients should receive more intense treatments. The best time to use moxa is early spring through early summer and from late summer into the fall.

1. Basic preventive moxibustion for patients with hypertension

Moxa *Zu San Li* (St 36) and *Xuan Zhong* (GB 39).[37] Many acupuncture texts do not mention that moxibustion may be applied to *Xuan Zhong*. Indeed, some Chinese doctors believe marrow points should not be heated. Nevertheless, this point is very effective for lowering blood pressure. Moxa cones work better than moxa rolls, since slight damage to the skin in this case is considered good. To heal the skin, a wash made from green onion, mint, peach leaf, or willow leaf tea is traditionally used.

2. Moxa "pens"

Multi-application point moxibustion "pens" burn two millimeter diameter moxa sticks indirectly on the body through a sandpaper-like sheet. Point moxibustion is performed by burning five dots on the sheet on each of various points on the body in the pattern of a pentagon. The recommended points are *Yang Ling Quan* (GB 34), *Zu San Li* (St 36), and *Feng Chi* (GB 20) which should be moxaed bilaterally. According to the instruction manual from the Shoumin Moxibustion Appliance Factory in Anhui, China, such moxibustion at these points can reduce systolic pressure by 20-30mmHg and diastolic pressure by 10-15mmHg with stable results.

3.

Moxa *Qu Chi* (LI 11), *Nei Guan* (Per 6), *Yang Ling Quan* (GB 34), and/or *San Yin Jiao* (Sp 6), depending on the patient's symptoms. Use 100 cones on *Guan Yuan* (CV 4), and teach the patient to use a moxa roll for 15 minutes per day in early winter.

4. Following a TIA

Preventive acupuncture therapy should be applied aggressively and as early as possible after a TIA. Even after years of TIA episodes, the following points have been found effective: *Ren Zhong* (GV 26), *Nei Guan* (Per 6), *San Yin Jiao* (Sp 6), *Ji Quan* (Ht 1), *Wei Zhong* (Bl 40), and *Chi Ze* (Lu 5). Needling these points has stopped the symptoms of TIA in 3-20 treatments in patients who had experienced TIAs for 2-20 years.[38]

5. For hypertension with arteriosclerosis

Acupuncture points and protocols addressing the TCM pattern of phlegm harassment have been found in research studies to help normalize blood pressure as well as effectively treat the initial stages of cerebral arteriosclerosis. For cases of hypertension with occlusion of the carotid artery, treat *Ren Ying* (St 9), *Fu Tu* (LI 18), *Qu Chi* (LI 11), and *Zu San Li* (St 36), adding *Nei Guan* (Per 6) and *Shen Men* (Ht 7) for agitation and insomnia. For relief of constipation, oliguria, restlessness, and a feeling of distention in the head, needle with moderate stimulation *Bai Hui* (GV 20), *Xuan Lu* (GB 5) or *Qu Bin* (GB 7), *Nei Guan* (Per 6), *Zu San Li* (St 36), and *San Yin Jiao* (Sp 6). If the patient's blood pressure is very high, strong needling stimulation should be avoided.[39]

6. Hypertension and syncope

According to Tran Viet Dzung, M.D., needling the window of the sky point *Ren Ying* (St 9) superficially directly over the carotid artery achieves good results in terms of lowering blood pressure. Dr. Tran has found that hypertension, vertigo, and syncope is sometimes due to an inability of the body to properly send qi downward to the lower part of the body. The lack of a pedal pulse indicates that qi is not descending properly. For this condition, Dr. Tran recommends needling together *Guan Yuan* (CV 4), *Heng Gu* (Ki 11) with superficial supplementation technique, *Qi Chong* (St 30) directed toward the foot, *Cheng Shan* (Bl 57), *Da Zhong* (Ki 4), *Chong Yang* (St 42), *Yong Quan* (Ki 1), *Da Dun* (Liv 1) located on dorsum of joint at hairs, *Gong Sun* (Sp 4), and *Nei Guan* (Per 6).

7. Hypertension

Fong Wan-Kei recommends the use of *Fu Tu* (LI 18) and *Ren Ying* (St 9) for the prevention of stroke. In a study, Dr. Fong treated 30 patients with hypertension and either the early signs of stroke, such as numbness of the tips of the fingers, headache with a pricking sensation, and stiff tongue, or with occlusion of the common carotid artery diagnosed by duplex carotid sonography. In addition to the above two points, Dr. Fong added *Qu Chi* (LI 11) and *Zu San Li* (St 36) on a routine basis. He also added *Qi Hai* (CV 6) and *Shen Men* (Ht 7) if there was agitation or insomnia. If there was profuse phlegm, he added *Tiao Kou* (St 38). The treatments used perpendicular needling once per day for 10 days, with 20-30 minutes' stimulation per treatment. The results showed an 87% total effectiveness rate, with 12 patients experiencing marked improvement, 14 cases experiencing some improvement, and four cases experiencing no effect.[40]

8. Hyperlipoproteinemia

According to Agnes Chen, clinical results from China suggest that acupuncture not only influences the metabolism of serum lipoprotein but also regulates serum lipoprotein ratios. *Zu San Li* (St 36), *Nei*

Guan (Per 6), and *San Yin Jiao* (Sp 6) have been used frequently in China to decrease serum lipoprotein levels within 20 treatments.[41] Acupuncture therapy has also been shown to regulate circulatory, digestive, and urinary system functions resulting in decreased hypertensive and hyperlipidemic states. In one study, *Gong Sun* (Sp 4), *San Yin Jiao* (Sp 6), *Qu Quan* (Liv 8), and *Zhong Wan* (CV 12) have been found to lower hyperlipoproteinemia. A second study using the same points with 86 hyperlipidemia patients found hyperlipoproteinemia types IIb and IV (WHO criteria) achieved the greatest decrease in values after 8-10 acupuncture treatments.[42] A 1990 study found that just needling at *Feng Long* (St 40) with a 1-1.5 inch needle decreased triglycerides notably after 20 treatments. Results from various studies indicate that *San Yin Jiao* (Sp 6), *Zu San Li* (St 36), and *Nei Guan* (Per 6) combined with *Tai Chong* (Liv 3) and *Feng Long* (St 40) are verifiably effective points for reducing hyperlipidemia.[43]

Preventing Stroke Through the Integration of Modern Western Medicine & Complementary Therapies

High blood pressure medication

It is well worth the effort to treat hypertension in any way acceptable to the patient. In patients with hypertension, even a partial reduction in blood pressure has been shown to decrease morbidity. Western pharmaceuticals are usually used to control blood pressure, but rapid control can also be gained with high doses of supplemental magnesium. Naturopathic doctors in the state of Washington are licensed to inject higher doses of magnesium than can be absorbed orally. Magnesium relaxes muscle tension, including the muscles that constrict blood vessels. Lifestyle intervention, such as diet modification or alcohol reduction, may substitute for medication or may enhance the medications' lowering of blood pressure.

More than just high cholesterol levels

Treating only those patients with high cholesterol levels overlooks 50% of people with atherosclerosis. With more screening tests using the same blood sample, we can know which specific lifestyle risk factor(s) are clogging the arteries of people with normal cholesterol levels. Doctors (particularly doctors who are skilled in evaluating the underlying lifestyle causes) can be consulted to monitor and interpret cholesterol levels. The range should be 180-200mg/dL. Low density lipids should be below 130mg/dL. Pre-menopausal women and women on hormone replacement therapy should have an HDL level above 50mg/dL, while men and post-menopausal women should have an HDL level above 40mg/dL. Everyone should have triglycerides (TG) below 140mg/dL. Consumer reports have evaluated five out of five home cholesterol tests and found them all to be lacking. But even professional laboratory cholesterol tests provide too little information.

According to research cardiologist Dr. Superko in *Before the Heart Attacks*, one half of the 1.5 million heart attacks in the United States strike people with "normal" cholesterol levels. Today, advanced metabolic markers can now be determined with a simple, inexpensive blood test to help this second 50% of people at risk for vascular disease. One of these tests measures the amount of so-called small LDL that is the most likely itself into the artery walls.

Small LDL is also statistically linked to high blood pressure. Small LDL measuring less than 257 angstroms in a concentration of 20% or above is of grave concern, relating to apolipoprotein B (Apo B) of 80mg/dL or above. Small LDL is also statistically linked to high blood pressure. The specific HDL subclass responsible for removing cholesterol from the arteries is HDL2B. HDL2B is the most strongly associated form of HDL with reduced risk of vascular disease. It should be above 35% in pre-menopausal women or women on hormone therapy and above 20% in men and postmenopausal women. C-reactive protein (CRP) should be 0.4mg/dL or below. Fibrinogen should be less than 400mg/dL. Chlamydia pneumoniae should be less than one part in 32, while insulin should be less than 12 mU/mL. Homocysteine should be less than 14 micromoles per liter, and lipoprotein (a) should be less than 20mg/dL. In addition, the presence of gene type apolipoprotein E2 or E4 indicates a patient's positive ability to respond to dietary changes in terms of reducing their vascular risk.

Top cardiologists researching the prevention of heart attack and stroke have developed a well-researched protocol for nutrition, exercise, medication, and supplements for each of the above metabolic markers. According to Dr. Superko, most atherosclerosis can be halted or reversed without drugs simply by the individualized nutritional and exercise regimens described in his book. However, medications like the statins, resins, fibrates, ezetimibe, aspirin, and niacin and supplements like fish oil, vitamin C, and vitamin E may also be essential for some patients.[44]

Help stopping smoking

All smokers who stop smoking reduce their *risk of ischemic stroke regardless of how much they previously smoked*, and there are medications, herbs, acupuncture, and support programs available to help smokers break their addiction. However, to get the most benefit, one should stop smoking as soon as possible. There are multiple health benefits from abstaining from smoking. One increasingly popular method to help stop smoking is auriculotherapy. This involves superficial needling of acupoints located in various positions on the external ear. Auriculotherapy can reduce a patient's physiological symptoms and psychological cravings while they quit smoking. However, self-motivation to stop is still required by the patient. One commonly used ear acupuncture smoking withdrawal protocol is to needle the Nicotine Point, Lung #1, Lung #2, Point Zero, Spirit Gate, Autonomic Point, and Ear Brain Point. Auxiliary points include Mouth, Adrenal Gland C, Adrenal Gland F, Aggression, and Limbic System points on the ear. Lung points can be treated with electroacupuncture at 80Hz for two minutes or simply needled for 20 minutes.[45]

CRP test

C-reactive protein testing is mostly of benefit to people with an intermediate risk of cardiovascular events—in other words, people with a 10-20% risk of such events in the next 10 years. To determine your risk level, ask your doctor or go to the Web site *http://hin.nhlbi. nih.gov/atpiii/calculator.asp?usertype=prof* . For people with an intermediate or moderate stroke risk, a more intense program of stroke prevention comprised of lowering blood pressure, quitting smoking, and eating healthier is indicated.[46] Elevated CRP levels appear to be associated with more unstable atherosclerotic plaque than lower CRP levels. Unstable plaque is more likely to rupture and lead to a stroke. So testing combined with appropriate treatment is crucial.

High body iron stores

High body iron stores may increase free radical production in brain cells, thus prompting stroke progression.[47] Treatments for hematochromatosis, a genetic condition of iron overload in the body, include blood donation and chelation therapy. See *www.drruhland.com* for information about chelation therapy.

Living a Healthy Lifestyle

The following suggestions all lead to living a healthier lifestyle and to reducing one's risk of stroke.

Control blood pressure

High blood pressure is the major risk factor in stroke. Thus it should be checked regularly and kept under control. Obesity, diabetes, alcohol intake, genetics, inactivity, and excess dietary sodium are all risk factors for hypertension. Nutritional magnesium deficiency should be addressed for adequate blood pressure control in addition to adequate and appropriate Western medication. As little as a 10-pound weight loss has been shown to decrease blood pressure in many overweight persons.[48] A recently published set of clinical trials called DASH (Dietary Approaches to Stop Hypertension) give the following guidelines to address blood pressure through dietary measures. The DASH diet is high in fruits and vegetables, fat-free or low-fat dairy products, whole grains, fish, poultry, and nuts. It reduces the amount of red meat and sweets. It is high in fiber, low in sodium, and includes minerals that we know contribute to lowered blood pressure, such as calcium,

magnesium, and potassium.[49]

Monitor blood pressure

Risk of stroke is increased for people if they discontinue hypertensive medication with a return of high blood pressure. This is because the artery walls are no longer adapted to the high pressure. Therefore, one should *not* discontinue medication permanently unless blood pressure stays close to the normal range. Be consistent with alternative therapies, and monitor blood pressure closely.

Keep track of all medications

It is important to keep track of all current medications. Maintain a minimum of a 3-day supply of medications in case of emergencies such as weather or a power failure were to limit access to a pharmacy.

Keep diabetes well controlled

Because high insulin levels cause unstable plaques to build in the arteries, it is important to keep blood sugar levels under good control. Exercise and good eating habits are the key to accomplishing this. Loss of weight, especially around the middle, reduces insulin resistance. Studies are still being conducted as to the best way to control blood sugar levels. Chinese medicine individualizes treatments and helps with weight loss, sleep, and blood sugar control. It also can help with pain to allow increased exercise.

Diet

Studies show that stroke risk is lowered by eating more whole grains and produce—especially leafy greens, citrus fruits, and cruciferous vegetables like broccoli, cabbage, and kale—and less red meat. In general, unsaturated fats are considerably better for us than are saturated fats. Of these, the omega-3's have the most protective qualities. Fish oils are the best source of omega-3's. Omega-6 fatty acids in oils such as corn, soybean, and safflower oils lower the good HDL and should not be used. Free-range, grass-fed animals are higher in essential omega-3 fatty acids than are grain-fed animals. Fats that decrease inflammation in the blood vessels include flax, fish, and olive oils. For cooking, use only olive oil, a monounsaturated fat, on low to moderate heat. Heating vegetable oils at high temperatures can change fatty acids and make them carcinogenic. Flax and fish oils should be taken cool in temperature such as in salad dressing. Hydrogenated vegetable oils, so-called trans fats, are well known to cause inflammation. They are still prevalent in most prepared foods since they are a cheap source of fat with a long shelf life. Thereforee, one should read package labels and avoid hydrogenated vegetable oil. Admittedly, this is impossible to do at restaurants. Hence food cooked at home with olive oil is the best. Olive oil is one of the few fats known to increase the HDL necessary for good cardiovascular function.

Sugars increase triglyceride levels. Even complex carbohydrate diets may result in high triglyceride levels because of the sheer volume of carbohydrates consumed.

In general, it is recommended to eat leaner cuts of meat and white-meat poultry since they are high in protein but relatively low in saturated fat. Although individuals react differently to dietary cholesterol, it is probably good to avoid high amounts.

Green leafy vegetables are high in B vitamins and are thus helpful to treat the enzyme deficiencies responsible for high homocysteine levels causing stroke. The American Heart Association recommends five daily servings of fruits and leafy green vegetables, broccoli, or beans.

Exercise, a most important prescription

A major factor in reducing stroke risk is daily exercise. Daily aerobic exercise to keep the heart rate up helps maintain healthy weight, lower blood pressure, improve cholesterol levels, control diabetes, and keep blood vessels flexible. Daily walking is recommended for the elderly or the sick. Qigong, meditation, and martial arts have been shown to reduce stroke risk in people with high blood pressure. A daily routine including work and rest, rising and going to bed early, and exercises that relax the body can help a patient recover from chronic stress. Only a few well designed longitudinal studies have associated stress with hypertension.[50] A large study in Sweden with 13,609 participants, mostly men, did find, however, that men who had suffered chronic stress had a 14% higher risk of heart attack and stroke even after adjusting the results for factors such as smoking and sedentary lifestyle. They also were twice as likely as their peers to die of a stroke.[51]

Providing enough time for deep sleep is essential

Weight-loss experts have a novel prescription for people who want to shed pounds: Get some sleep. In a study of approximately 18,000 adults, a strong link was found between the amount of sleep people get and their risk of becoming obese. Those who got less than four hours of sleep a night were 73% more likely to be obese than those who got the recommended 7-9 hours of rest. Those who averaged five hours of sleep had 50% greater risk, and those who got six hours had 23% more risk.

Specialists think that chronic sleep deprivation affects the body's food-seeking circuitry and may be what makes the difference in obesity risk. Sleep deprivation lowers leptin, a blood protein that suppresses appetite and seems to affect how the brain senses when the body has had enough food. Sleep deprivation also raises levels of grehlin, a substance that makes people want to eat.[52]

Additional Nutritional Therapies to Reduce Stroke Risk

Doctors and practitioners who have additional training in nutritional therapies have many tools for preventing strokes. The following are some of the therapies available.

Red yeast extract

Red yeast rice has been found to lower total cholesterol, raise HDL, and lower triglyceride levels.[53] A UCLA study published in the *American Journal of Clinical Nutrition* in 1999 reported that, after 12 weeks of red yeast rice supplementation, cholesterol levels among the 79 participants decreased by 15%. Red yeast rice works like the "statin" drugs Lipitor® and Zocor® by inhibiting a key liver enzyme from producing cholesterol. Naturopaths and Chinese doctors have used it for years to lower cholesterol. Research thus far has shown that red yeast rice does not carry with it the side effects associated with the pharmaceutical statin drugs. However, recently the FDA banned red yeast rice from over-the-counter sales because of the statins found naturally therein and valid concerns over liver damage. Alternatives, like policosanol and the B vitamin niacin, exist.

Niacin

Niacin or nicotinic acid positively effects all cholesterol abnormalities.[54] This vitamin is inexpensive and has been used to treat lipid disorders for decades. It has also been the subject of many successful studies that have demonstrated improved heart disease outcomes. In addition, niacin is relatively safe. Nevertheless, it should be taken under a doctor's supervision. This is because liver enzymes should be monitored if high therapeutic doses of niacin are required. Sustained-release niacin formulas have incurred problems. Niacin is contraindicated with liver disorders, gout, or high blood pressure.[55] Niacin combined with fibrates raise HDL levels in two different ways. Niacin combined with lower doses of statin drugs can be very successful at reducing atherosclerosis with fewer of the side effects than high-dose statins alone.[56]

Antioxidants

Antioxidants are helpful for people with high levels of small LDL, high triglycerides, high Lp(a), low HDL2B, and for people who smoke.[57] A person's risk of stroke is reduced if he or she takes the typical dose of natural vitamin E contained in a multivitamin supplement each day.[58] Impaired endothelium-dependent vasodilation (EDV) in diabetes type I can be improved by long-term administration of oral antioxidants (1000mg vitamin C and 800IU natural vitamin E).[59] High doses of natural vitamin E have been shown to decrease LDL peroxidation in persons under oxidative stress. The consumption of food products containing moderate amounts of vitamin E and carotenoids can lead to measurable and significant improvements in antioxidant status and biomarkers of oxidative stress in healthy persons as well.[60] Some recent research has found problems with high doses of vitamin E, but these problems may have been due to the nature of the synthetic vitamin as opposed to its natural form.

Omega-3 oils

Omega-3 oils can reduce stroke risk with fewer side effects than the drugs policosanol and aspirin. Studies are beginning to show that consumption of cold-water fish reduces the incidence of clotting stroke without the increase in hemorrhagic stroke. People with high triglycerides and high blood pressure, people with a large amount of small LDLs, and people with existing coronary heart disease should take 3-6 grams of fish oil per day.[61] More fish oil may be necessary. The advice of a physician keeping track of the disease progression with IMT carotid ultrasound and the advanced metabolic marker tests should be sought in this matter. Some doctors prescribe the drugs policosanol and aspirin which work synergistically to inhibit the formation of clots. However, if there is a risk of hemorrhagic stroke, policosanol and aspirin should be avoided. Udo Oil, a blend of oils developed by Dr. Udo, has helped some people's good HDL levels increase immensely. The best researched source of omega-3 oil is fish and fish oil.

Folic acid

Folic acid intake of at least 300 micrograms per day reduced the risk of stroke by 20% compared with consumption of less than 136 micrograms of folic acid or folate per day.[62] The Greek origin of the word folate means "leafy green." Leafy, dark green vegetables like spinach and chard are high in folic acid and have countless beneficial properties.[63]

Coffee

Coffee, including decaffeinated coffee, which contains significant amounts of the clotting factor vitamin K, should be avoided if one is at risk of ischemic stroke.

Serum copper levels

A copper deficiency has been associated with weakening of connective tissue that can be a contributing factor for hemorrhagic stroke. Copper is a heavy metal necessary only in small amounts. Wearing a copper bracelet ensures that only a nontoxic amount of copper is absorbed by the body.

Other Possibly Useful Vitamins and Herbs

The amino acid taurine as well as vitamin B6 reduce platelet aggregation. Eicosapentanoic acid (EPA) and high doses of omega-3 oils reduce platelet aggregation. Botanical remedies like garlic, cayenne pepper (Capsicum frutescens), ginkgo biloba, gugulipids, and turmeric extract (curcumin) are all alleged to reduce platelet aggregation.

Chelation therapy

Chelation therapy uses nutritional supplementation or intravenous injection of substances that bind with problematic substances in the body that cause narrowing of blood vessels. These problematic substances are then able to be excreted from the body. Chelation therapy is most helpful after the blood lipids have been well controlled.

Vegetarian or vegan diets

Wherever fresh vegetable consumption is high, there is a low incidence of cerebrovascular disease and thus fewer strokes.

Conclusion

Reducing the risks of stroke is a great deal less painful and less costly than suffering the rehabilitation from stroke, especially if a common-sense approach is taken. Noninvasive carotid IMT ultrasound can determine in what way and to what degree arteries are clogged. Blood pressure can and should be controlled. New blood tests are better at determining each individual's best therapies for decreasing atherosclerosis. People at low risk for stroke and with no changes in how they feel can prevent stroke simply with healthy meals, regular exercise, and regular sleep. We all know people who have entire cupboards full of drugs and supplements. These are often not necessary. As stroke risk rises, sensible professionals exist to help people find (and be consistent with) the exercise and diet prescriptions and remedies that are most effective and cost-effective for them as individuals. This is compassionate care.

Endnotes

[1] Appel, Lawrence, MD, & Elinas, Rafael, MD, "Hypertension and Stroke," *The John Hopkins White Papers,* Baltimore, MD, 2005, p. 45-50

[2] P-I News Services, "Morning Blood Pressure May Predict Stroke Risk," *Seattle Post-Intelligencer,* 2003, March 4, *www.seattlepi.com*

[3] Hajjar, I & Kotchen, T.A., "Trends in Prevalence, Awareness, Treatment, and Control of Hypertension in the United States, 1988-2000," *JAMA,* 2003; 290, p. 199, as cited in Wesa, KM & Grimm, R.H., "Recommendations and Guidelines Regarding the Preferred Research Protocol for Investigating the Impact of an Optimal Healing Environment on Patients with Hypertension," *The Journal of Alternative and Complementary Medicine,* 2004, 21 Supplement 1, p. S-246

[4] Superko, Robert H. & Tucker, Laura, *Before the Heart Attacks,* Plume, Penguin Group, NY 2003, p. 70

[5] *Ibid.,* p. 52

[6] Appel, *op. cit.,* p. 48

[7] Aldoori, Munther I & Rahman, Sakhawat, "Smoking and Stroke: A Causative Role," *BMJ,*

1998; 317, p. 962

[8] Kurth, T *et al.,* "Smoking and the Risk of Hemorrhagic Stroke in Men," *Stroke,* 2003, May; 34(5), p. 1151

[9] Motoyama, Takeshi *et al.,* "Endothelium-dependent Vasodilation in the Brachial Artery is Impaired in Smokers: Effect of Vitamin C," *American Journal of Physiology—Heart and Circulatory Physiology,* 1997; 273, p. H1644-H1650,

[10] Niskanen, Leo *et al.,* "Carotid Artery Intima-Media Thickness in Elderly Patients With NIDDM and in Nondiabetic Subjects," *Stroke,* 1996; 27, p. 1986

[11] Appel, *op. cit.,* p. 48-49

[12] Greenland, Philip *et al.,* "Prevention Conference V: Beyond Secondary Prevention: Identifying the High-Risk Patient for Primary Prevention," *Circulation,* 2000; 101, p. 111

[13] Honda, Osamu *et al.,* "Echolucent Carotid Plaques Predict Future Coronary Events in Patients with Coronary Artery Disease," *J Am Coll Cardiol,* 2004;43, p. 1177

[14] Author not cited. "Treating A Hidden Cause of Stroke," *The John Hopkins Medical Letter,* 1996, March, p. 3

[15] Reynoles, Kristi, *et al.,* "Alcohol Consumption and Risk for Stroke, A Meta-analysis," *JAMA,* 2003; 289, p. 579

[16] Kreeger, Karen, "Penn Researchers Add More Evidence To Demonstrate the Role of COX Inhibitors in Heart Disease Risk," University of Pennsylvania Medical Center, 2005, Jan 17, *http://www.uphs.upenn.edu/news/ News_Releases/jan05/COX.htm*

[17] Appel, *op. cit.,* p. 48

[18] *Ibid.,* p. 48

[19] Superko & Tucker, *op. cit.,* p. 235

[20] Appel, *op. cit.,* p. 48

[21] Author not cited, University of Washington 2005,*http://www.uwmedicine.org/uwmed/Templa tes/content/uwmedicine_storyNoContact.aspx?N RMODE=Published&NRORIGINALURL=%2fF acilities%2fHarborview%2fClinicsAndServices %2fNeuro%2fStrokeCenter%2fterms%2ehtm&N RNODEGUID=%7bBB3356FB-523B-4031-9B093C5FBFECDFCF%7d&NRCACHEHINT= Guest#top*

[22] Appel, *op. cit.,* p. 48

23 *Ibid.*, p. 44-46

24 *Ibid.*, p. 46

25 *Ibid.*, p. 46

26 Ruland, S. *et al.,* "Awareness, Treatment, and Control of Vascular Risk Factors in African Americans with Stroke," *Neurology*, 2003, Jan 14; 60(1), p. 64

27 Appel, *op. cit.*, p. 44

28 *Ibid.*, p. 44

29 *Ibid,.* p. 44

30 *Ibid.*, p. 44

31 Cheng Hai *et al.*, *Stroke*, China TCM Publishing, Beijing, China, 1995, p. 120-121

32 *Ibid.*, p. 122-13, and Shi Yu-guang *et al., Well-Known Physician's Clinical Experience in Present—-Stroke*, Classic TCM Book Publisher, Beijing, China, 1999, p. 264-265

33 *Ibid.*, p. 264-265 and Cheng, *op. cit.*, p. 120-121

34 Liu Bing-quan, "Prevention of Stroke," *Sing Tao News*, San Francisco, 1994, May 18, p. B5

35 Chen, Agnes, "Effective Acupuncture Therapy for Stroke and Cerebrovascular Diseases-Part III: Prescription for Prevention," *American Journal of Acupuncture*, 1993, Vol.21, No.4, p. 313

36 Tian Cong-hua *et al.*, *Chinese Moxibustion Experienced Collection*, Liaoning Scientific & Technical Publishing, Shenyang, China, 1987, p. 161-163

37 *Ibid.*,p. 161

38 Chen, *op. cit.*, p. 307

39 *Ibid.*, p. 310

40 Fong, Wan-Kei, *Compilation of the Abstracts of Acupuncture and Moxibustion Papers*, The First World Conference of Acupuncture-Moxibustion, Acupuncture Medicine Association of Southern California, p. 38

41 Chen, *op. cit.*, p. 311

42 *Ibid.*, p. 311

43 *Ibid.*, p. 311

44 Superko & Tucker, *op. cit.*, p. 248-251

45 Oleson, Terry, *Auriculotherapy Manual: Chinese and Western Systems of Ear Acupuncture*, Second Edition, Health Care Alternatives, Los Angeles, CA, 1996, p. 182

46 No author cited, "C-Reactive Protein: A New Risk Factor for Stroke," *Hypertension and Stroke, www.HopkinsAfter50.com*, 2004

47 Davalos, A. *et al.*, "Body Iron Stores and Early Neurologic Deterioration in Acute Cerebral Infarction," *Neurology*, 2000; 54, p. 1568

48 Wesa, K.M. & Grimm, R.H., *op.cit.*, p. S-246

49 Superko & Tucker, *op. cit.*, p. 156

50 Wesa & Grimm, *op.cit.*, p. S-246

51 Ohlin B, *et al.*, "Chronic Psychosocial Stress Predicts Long-term Cardiovascular Morbidity and Mortality in Middle-aged Men," *European Heart Journal*, 2004, May; 25(10), p. 867

52 Heymsfield, Steven & Gangwisch, James, *Meeting of the North American Association for the Study of Obesity.* "Presenting a Study Linking Sleep Deprivation and Obesity," November 14-18, 2004

53 "Chinese Cholesterol Cure?" *HealthNews*, June 24, 1997, p. 6

54 "Update on Cholesterol and Red Yeast Rice," *www.wholehealthmd.com*

55 Balch, Phyllis A. & Balch, James F. *Prescription for Nutritional Healing,* Third ed., Avery Publishing, New York, 2000, p. 441

56 Superko & Tucker, *op. cit.*, p. 265-276

57 *Ibid.* p.291

58 Benson, Richard, "Vitamin E may reduce risk of stroke," 51st Meeting of the American Academy of Neurology

59 Beckman, Joshua A, *et al.*, "Oral Antioxidant Therapy Improves Endothelial Function in Type 1 but Not Type 2 Diabetes Mellitus," *American Journal of Physiology & Heart Circulatory Physiology*, 2003, 285, p. H2392

60 Upritchard, Jane E. *et al.*, "Spread Supplemented with Moderate Doses of Vitamin E and Carotenoids Reduces Lipid Peroxidation in Healthy, Nonsmoking Adults," *American Journal of Clinical Nutrition,* November 2003, Vol.78, No.5, p. 985

61 Superko & Tucker, *op. cit.,* p. 297

62 *Stroke,* 2002; 33, p. 1183-9

63 Lamphere, Karen, "The Virtues of Greens," *PCC Sound Consumer*, July 2005, No. 83, p. 1

APPENDIX ONE
The Chinese National Standard for the Diagnosis of Stroke & Outcomes of its Treatment

In 1978, the Second All National Congress on Neurology & Psychiatry was held in Nanjing to help create the following standard of diagnostic criteria for clinical trials dealing with strokes and their therapeutic outcomes. Since then within the People's Republic of China, all practitioners treating stroke patients (whether modern Western or traditional Chinese medical doctors) are required to use the following criteria for definitions, diagnostic labels, and the assessment of outcomes.[1]

A. The classification of acute symptoms

1. Ischemic type

a. Transient ischemic attack (TIA)

1. A very short and reversible attack caused by poor cerebrovascular circulation. It is also recurrent with one-two or even more than a hundred attacks. It is mostly related to cerebral arteriosclerosis, and it may be the warning sign of arteriothrombosis with brain infarction.

2. Symptoms and physical signs of ischemic infarction of the internal carotid artery and basilar artery may appear.

3. The duration of each attack lasts for a few minutes to one hour, and all symptoms and physical signs disappear within 24 hours.

b. Cerebral thrombosis

1. Symptoms appear more often while the patient is in a calm condition.

2. Most of the time this condition is not accompanied by severe hematopathy, headache, or vomiting.

3. Onset is relatively slow with gradual worsening of the condition. Most of the time it is related to cerebral arteriosclerosis. Sometimes it can be accompanied by vasculitis, leptospirosis, or hematopathy.

4. Patient stays conscious or their consciousness is only slightly disturbed during the onset of the disease, *i.e.*, one-two days.

5. Six hours after onset, there is usually no blood in the spinal fluid.

6. Patient shows the symptoms of ischemia of the internal carotid artery and basilar artery. The sclerosis on the internal carotid artery may be classified as five types: acute (stroke), recurrent, chronic, dementia-form, and asymptomatic. The symptoms of sclerosis of the basilar artery are a sudden loss of consciousness resembling Meniere's syndrome of the subclavian artery and imperforation.

c. Cerebral embolism

1. Acute onset

2. Normally no prominent symptoms.

3. Patient can be conscious with a temporary disturbance of consciousness.

4. Six hours after the onset, the spinal fluid should be checked to make sure that there is no blood in the fluid.

5. Patient shows the symptoms relating to the supply zone of the carotid artery and basilar artery.

6. The embolism may or may not be from the heart. It is possible to show infarction of other organs, skin, or bulbar conjunctiva.

2. Hemorrhagic type

a. Intracranial hemorrhage

The majority of intracranial hemorrhage is from hypertension caused by arterial sclerosis. It may include other hemorrhaging; it is not caused by injury.

1. Onset occurs most often during physical exercise or emotional tension.

2. Patient has recurrent vomiting and headache.

3. Symptoms may get worse rapidly;

unconsciousness, paralysis or other neurological symptoms may appear.

4. Most often, patient has hypertension and cranial artery sclerosis.

5. 85-90% will show blood in the spinal fluid exam.

6. May see positive changes in ultrasound exam.

b. Subarachnoid hemorrhage

The majority of subarachnoid hemorrhages happen in broken congenital malformations and in sclerosis of the cranial artery.

1. Sudden onset of symptoms. Young cases are mostly caused by an aneurysm. Older than middle-age cases are more likely to be caused by sclerosis of the artery.

2. Often have severe headache and vomiting.

3. Signs of neurological damage to cerebrum and paralysis may appear.

4. Patient may be conscious with light disturbance of consciousness and mental disorder.

5. Blood appears in the spinal fluid.

6. Requires cerebral angiography for accurate diagnosis.

B. A four-fold division of standard treatment outcomes

1. Basically cured

The motor function of the paralytic extremity is basically recovered. Myodynamia is improved to four-five degrees, and the patient can take care of him- or herself. Any facial paralysis and speech problems have disappeared.

2. Markedly effective

The motor function of the paralytic extremity shows a marked recovery. Myodynamia reaches four degrees or improves by three degrees. Facial paralysis is markedly improved. Patient is basically able to take care of him- or herself.

3. Improved

The motor function of the extremity is improved. Myodynamia has improved by one degree, but the patient still cannot walk without assistance.

4. No effect

After treatment, the patient's symptoms remain unchanged.

Endnote

[1] No author cited, "A Plan For the Prevention & Treatment of Cerebral Vascular Disease," *Zhong Hua Shen Jing Jing Shen Ke Za Zhi (Chinese Journal of Neurology & Psychiatry),* #2, 1978, p. 127

APPENDIX TWO
Acupuncture in Post-stroke Rehabilitation: Functional & Neuroplastic Considerations by Kathleen Michael, Ph.D., RN, CRRN

In the United States of America, stroke is the greatest cause of disability in adults. Advances in emergency care have resulted in improved survival rates and increasing numbers of people who live with disability in the aftermath of strokes. The majority of stroke survivors have disability that affects self-care, mobility, communication, or social function. Thus there is an imperative to improve function, independence, and quality of life in stroke survivors. The application of acupuncture in stroke rehabilitation is appropriate to this goal.

Acupuncture is an effective treatment following stroke but is not widely used in America. Complementary therapies, such as acupuncture and herbal medicine, are not routinely included in post-stroke rehabilitation for a variety of reasons. First, the basic principles of traditional Chinese medicine are not well understood by Western health care providers. Following the mechanistic, disease-oriented medical model, Western health care providers emphasize treatment of pathology and development of compensatory strategies for existing disability rather than promoting the body's own heal-

ing capacities as mediated by the balance of qi. These are very different world views. Yet there are links and similarities, particularly relative to stroke, that may inform the practice of rehabilitation medicine and warrant thoughtful exploration and application.

Second, health care in America is strongly driven by economics, and financial coverage of acupuncture services as part of a rehabilitation program is seldom supported by insurance and managed care resources. There is a need to demonstrate that the actual outcomes of acupuncture treatment in stroke recovery reduce health care costs, particularly in terms of functional recovery and independence and reduction in sequelae and co-morbidities that drive up healthcare resource utilization. Solid, objective evidence that acupuncture is an effective treatment for stroke and that it results in lower health care costs is needed to propel change in the industry and convince providers to integrate acupuncture into rehabilitation practice.

Third, there are not enough partnerships between Western and Chinese medicine practitioners so that the treatments can be coordinated and implemented seamlessly and in a timely fashion in the context of American medicine to result in the greatest improvement for stroke survivors. While it is ideal to incorporate acupuncture as soon as possible following stroke, it is not widely integrated into acute stroke care and may only be considered when other therapy options have been exhausted. As emphasized in this text, the sooner acupuncture treatment is begun following stroke, the more effective it is.

Further, when patients no longer make progressive functional improvements after their strokes, they often cease to receive therapy benefits. The notion of a "plateau" in stroke recovery, signaling the end of the recovery process, is implicated in short-changing the potential of many stroke patients. Many classic measurements of functional improvement fail to capture elements that would indicate potential for further recovery. By discontinuing therapy services, the fate of stroke patients is sealed, and their failure to progress after the first three to six months may have more to do with loss of treatment than with an actual end to recovery potential. Studies at the Claude D. Pepper Center at the University of Maryland have shown that neuroplastic changes can be induced months and years after the occurrence of stroke, suggesting that the capacity for recovery is not time-limited. It is possible that acupuncture facilitates the natural processes that produce new or enhanced areas of activation in the brain as evidenced by similar patterns of recovery demonstrated in Chinese studies.

Rehabilitation is extremely valuable in maximizing mobility and self-care and in developing compensatory strategies for specific deficits. But, conventional rehabilita-

tion only starts the recovery process. Typically, post-stroke rehabilitation consists of about 10-14 days of intense therapy (physical, occupational, speech), followed by approximately eight weeks of either home or out patient therapies delivered approximately three times per week. These therapies are discontinued when progress slows. Many patients and families are told and many care providers believe that whatever recovery patients experience in the first three-six months after stroke is all that can be expected. While the failure to make continued functional gains in recovery is often attributed to the nature and effects of the stroke, it is possible that the plateau in recovery is actually related to the finite provision of therapies and not to the inherent capacity for recovery that persists through life.

There is reason to take full advantage of the window of recovery and not be limited by the traditionally accepted time frames. As demonstrated in many studies described in this book, acupuncture is effective months and years after the stroke. This may relate to the concept that the capacity for neuroplastic change may be leveraged toward functional improvements after stroke by directing specific treatments and actions. Acupuncture, particularly coupled with movement and exercise, may play a role in motor learning and neuroplasticity responses.

Acupuncture is also known to be effective in controlling function-limiting symptoms, such as spasticity. When such symptoms are relieved, patients may be able to use their residual function to greater advantage. By practicing movements and functional activities under conditions of less limitation, patients can develop range of motion, strength, endurance, and motor learning leading to improvements in independence and self-care. Here is where the combination of acupuncture and Western rehabilitation may work in synergy to the functional benefit of stroke patients.

The dramatic observations that have been reported following acupuncture treatment that combine movement with needling give credence to the possibility that acupuncture along with physical movement may enhance the neuroplastic response. Further research is needed to map the brain activity and identify the specific response to acupuncture treatments, but the strong evidence of the effectiveness of acupuncture, even after other therapies have ceased to demonstrate improvement, cannot be dismissed. The opportunity exists to couple acupuncture with established Western methods of rehabilitation toward increased function, independence, and quality of life for stroke survivors.

APPENDIX THREE
My Experiences with Acupuncture Treating Neurological Conditions
by Craig M. Brewer, M.D. (General Practice & Family Medicine)

I had long since been convinced of and had firsthand experience in using acupuncture to treat painful conditions in my patients. In 1984, a 25-year-old man came into my medical clinic with severe spasticity in his arm and hand secondary to a gun shot wound that had grazed the nerve root of C6 in his neck. I was in a quandary of how to treat him. My acupuncturist, Hoy Ping Yee Chan (who worked with me in my office at that time), said that acupuncture might help him. I said, "This is a neuromuscular (motor) condition," and asked if acupuncture could help spasticity. She said, "Yes, acupuncture is used frequently in China for paralysis and related conditions."

With the patient's consent, Dr. Chan inserted about eight needles on the selected acupoints. Manual manipulation of the needles was applied and the needles were retained for 20 minutes. With this initial treatment, my patient was able to fully open his fisted hand in three-four seconds. Prior to this treatment and since his injury several months before, the fastest he could open his hand was in about 15 seconds and, even then, it was not completely open.

This dramatic improvement in spasticity was sustained when he came in for follow up treatment in two days. At that time, his only complaint was muscle pain in his forearm, *i.e.*, in the muscles that were able to be fully used for the first time in several months. Subsequently, I have treated and witnessed improvement in motor spasticity caused from spinal cord trauma to head trauma, strokes and other CNS pathology.

As for an explanation of the mechanism of action, afferent input from acupuncture needling may stimulate centers in the brainstem that tone down spastic efferent impulses originating in damaged higher motor areas of the brain.

The time frame for acupuncture intervention for the stroke patient is of critical importance. As with any modality considered in the treatment of illness, once a disease process has settled in for six months or more it is difficult to show much further improvement no matter what treatment one chooses.

In stroke treatment there is also an observation

period from the time since onset (TSO) of the neurological event before one should consider initiating therapy, including acupuncture. It takes from a few to several days to sort out what and how much of a neurological deficit will remain.

If a patient is rapidly improving they may not need any intervention. On the other hand, if a patient has a dense flaccid paralysis, acupuncture would be futile (as would any other modality) until such time that the paralysis may improve from flaccid to spastic (say over the first two-four weeks) and then be amenable to acupuncture's ability to treat spasticity.

A good timing for starting acupuncture in stroke may be at the time a patient is transferred to rehabilitation from an acute care hospital, approximately one-two weeks TSO. This group of patients is not only in the correct time frame for starting intensive rehabilitation training and modalities, but (if qualified for rehabilitation) have the potential for meaningful improvement. They also have enough deficits to need therapy, in which acupuncture could play a significant role.

Thus I believe it is timely that this book has arrived that presents a current and comprehensive description of the use of acupuncture for stroke and other motor disorders.

APPENDIX FOUR
Patients & Their Families Talking About Stroke

Stroke can be devastating for both the patient and his or her family. The toll it takes on the physical and emotional health of all involved can be monumental. I have seen many stroke patients in my practice. Many have high spirits and struggle to create an independent life and full recovery while receiving their acupuncture treatments. I have been deeply impressed by their actions and attitudes in the face of adversity.

Trust and confidence in acupuncture therapy and in the practitioner are very important to keep stroke patients coming for regular treatments and following the prescribed treatment plan. Patients and their family members have to make a commitment to work towards the goal of recovery together. This is the key to successful rehabilitation.

Timberly, the son of one of my stroke patients, is very supportive of his disabled mother. His wonderful spirit and good attitude deeply impressed me. Although his mother presented a difficult case to treat, the commitment between her, her husband, her son and myself, worked well in helping

her to gain a reasonable recovery. What follows is Timberly's thoughts about this process.

Holistic Approach to the Treatment of Stroke

"Victims of stroke suffer spiritually and emotionally as well as physically. Loved ones suffer with the victim, as relationships are affected by the well-being of those involved in these relationships. Family members love and depend upon each other. Instinctively family members want to help stroke victims recover as fully and quickly as the victims themselves [do]. Patients and caregivers should seek as many resources as possible, to achieve as much recovery as possible. I want to share some sources beyond the traditional stroke therapy that would help other stroke victims and their caregivers. Our family has learned to appreciate the many blessings of our situation and has had the good fortune to find many more in over four years of experiencing mother's stroke recovery. Learning from other stroke victims, their families, the Stroke Association, therapists, physicians, and mother's acupuncturist, we have come to appreciate several important things that could help others. First, and most important, is spiritual strength. Whatever the source of spiritual faith is, regardless of religious background, it is important for the patient and those who care for the patient to nurture and encourage their spiritual well being. Faith gives people strength, hope, patience, and persistence. The absence of faith leads to despair and the loss of the will-power necessary to continue the daily struggle towards recovery. Depression and despondency compound recovery problems. Losing so many things of such importance, knowing they may be gone forever, and facing such a long and hard road to recovery, it seems easier to give up. But it is a dark and miserable life to do nothing and waste away. Spiritual health gives us emotional strength. Again, determination and persistence are essential to maintain the motivation to exercise and persevere. Resentment at loss of communication, motor skills, and mental ability is as vicious an adversary as the physical disabilities themselves. This affects the victim most severely, but it also affects family members and care-givers."

"Emotional strength provides the persistence required for rehabilitation exercises. Just as we develop any skills, those lost to stroke must be painfully regained through meticulous practice. Physical, occupational, speech therapy and exercises have to be done over and over again, day after day. The motivation to keep up with an exercise program depends on the emotional strength of the stroke victim and the encouragement of caregivers. The patient's acceptance and willingness are the first steps to the perseverance that will be required to achieve recovery. What we call traditional stroke treatment leaves out an important part of the stroke victim's treatment. Traditional

stroke therapy is based on physiology and physiological function. With this focus, Western medicine addresses the most obvious afflictions. However, the whole being is not treated. Oriental medicine provides treatment for more subtle and powerful, equally important aspects of the patient, areas that Western medicine cannot easily improve."

"Working in concert with traditional therapy, acupuncture can help in a complementary and synergistic manner to improve the rate and degree of recovery in many cases. Acupuncture can provide the greatest help if treatment is sought and applied as soon after the stroke as the acupuncturist and physician believe is appropriate. However, acupuncture is not a "quick fix" and requires repeated treatments. The persistence and patience that are required from those seeking treatment are also required of those providing the treatment. It takes a special kind of practitioner, one willing to spend the time that stroke victim's need, to do the things that the practitioner used to do in an instant. The acupuncturist must also have the time and patience that different methods require. I deeply admire my mother's spiritual faith and my father's endless love. I also admire Dr. Chan for her treatment of stroke patients. She gives ample time and her complete attention to every patient according to each one's individual needs."

"Through the continued pursuit of acupuncture treatment, my mother has received many specific benefits. She first sought treatment for disabling chronic pain, and felt relief after her first treatment. After the source of the pain was finally found and corrected, Dr. Chan was able to focus on helping to further mother's stroke rehabilitation. I should point out that mother had been discharged by therapists, yet knew she could achieve more full recovery. She continued to experience edema in her affected leg after a fall. However, this was reduced with acupuncture. Dr. Chan's treatments to improve circulation also helped mother's general health which led to better strength and the courage to try more advanced rehabilitation methods. Dr. Chan included scalp and eye techniques that produced remarkable improvement in mother's walking and speech."

"I strongly urge stroke victims and their families to seek acupuncture treatment. Do not wait, nor consider acupuncture to simply be a last resort or only for pain relief. Most insurers do not cover acupuncture, but many agencies and social services can help in some way. It is the responsibility of the patient and family to continue further recovery. An open mind and willingness to try acupuncture will allow stroke victims the opportunity to see for themselves how they can benefit from treatments. I also challenge therapists and physicians to learn how acupuncture can benefit their patients and encourage acupuncturists to continue to learn more advanced techniques, like Dr. Chan."

(Written by Timberly Links, C.P.A.)

Another stroke survivor adds the following comments about her experience with acupuncture:

"After my stroke, physical therapy helped me get back on my feet, but it was limited in its effectiveness. I felt that I was getting stronger over time, but I also was getting less flexible. The rigidity or "tone" in my arm and leg were not improving with strengthening exercises. I began to try relaxation techniques and meditation which helped increase the functioning of my affected limbs."

"A number of people suggested that I try acupuncture in order to support my recovery. I resisted their advice because I was unfamiliar with acupuncture and I was afraid it would be painful. Finally, I did try acupuncture, and, although it was quite a while after my stroke, I felt significant improvement in a short time. My limbs felt more flexible. My circulation improved. I was able to do activities which I had not been able to do for a long time, such as walking my dog and washing my hair with both hands! My only regret is that I did not begin treatment sooner. I wish that all stroke survivors had access to the benefits of acupuncture."

(Written by Ms. Y.)

English Language Bibliography

This bibliography only lists the English language books and articles used in the preparation of this book. Bibliographic information on the many Chinese language books and articles used in the research for this book are listed in the endnotes of each individual chapter in which they appear. Within this bibliography, journal and Web site articles are separated from book titles.

Journal & Web site articles

"A Special Needling Technique," Lu Shou-kang *et al.*, *One Hundred Techniques of Acupuncture*, China Medical Science, Beijing, China, First Edition, Oct. 1987

"A Study Linking Sleep Deprivation and Obesity," Steven Heymsfield & James Gangwisch, Meeting of the North American Association for the Study of Obesity, November 14-18, 2004

"Alcohol Consumption and Risk for Stroke: A Meta-analysis," Kristi Reynolds *et al.*, *Journal of the American Medical Association*, 2003; 289, p. 579

"Awareness, Treatment, and Control of

Vascular Risk Factors in African Americans with Stroke," S. Ruland *et al.*, *Neurology*, 2003, Jan. 14; 60(1), p. 64

"Body Iron Stores and Early Neurologic Deterioration in Acute Cerebral Infarction," A. Davalos *et al.*, *Neurology,* 2000; 54, p. 1568

"C-Reactive Protein: A New Risk Factor for Stroke," No author cited, *Hypertension and Stroke,* 2004, www.HopkinsAfter50.com.

"Carotid Artery Intima-Media Thickness in Elderly Patients With NIDDM and in Nondiabetic Subjects," Leo Niskanen *et al.*, *Stroke,* 1996; 27, p. 1986

"Change in Motor Unit Synchronization Following Central Nervous Lesions in Man," S. F. Farmer *et al.*, *Journal of Physiology*, No. 463, p. 83-105

"Chinese Cholesterol Cure?" No author cited, *HealthNews*, June 24, 1997, p. 6

"Chronic Psychosocial Stress Predicts Long-term Cardiovascular Morbidity and

Mortality in Middle-aged Men," B. Ohlin *et al.*, *European Heart Journal,* 2004 May; 25(10), p. 867

"Clinical Application of the 3 Tongue-Points in Aphasia," Lai Xin-sheng, *International Journal of Clinical Acupuncture*, New York, 1999, Vol. 10, No. 2, p. 185-187

"CT Scanning and Therapeutic Effects of Acupuncture on 108 Cases of Hemiplegia Due to Apoplexy," Fang Yuan *et al.*, *International Journal of Clinical Acupuncture*, New York, 1990, Vol. 1, No. 1, p. 1-6

"Developing a Research Strategy for the Acupuncture Professional: Research Questions, Resources Necessary to Answer Them, and Guidelines for Matching Resources to Types of Research, Clinical Acupuncture, and Oriental Medicine," Stephen Birch, Ph.D., L.Ac. *et al.,* title of publication, Elsevier Science Ltd. Amsterdam, 2003, Volume 4, Issue 1, p. 29-33, *A Practical Dictionary of Chinese Medicine*, Nigel Wiseman & Feng Ye, Paradigm Publications, Brookline, MA, 1998

"Diagnostic Imaging in Diagnosis of Stroke," Robert C. Goigney, MD, Current Advances in Stroke Symposium, Seattle, WA, June 19, 1986

"Dysfuncton of Upper Limbs as Sequela of Stroke Treated with T-Shaped Needling," Liu Zhen-chun, *International Journal of Clinical Acupuncture,* New York, 1995, Vol. 6, No. 1, p. 73-74

"Echolucent Carotid Plaques Predict Future Coronary Events in Patients with Coronary Artery Disease," Osamu Honda *et al.*,

Journal of the American College of Cardiology, 2004; 43, p. 1177

"Effective Acupuncture Therapy for Stroke and Cerebrovascular Diseases, Part III: Prescription for Prevention," Agnes Chen, *American Journal of Acupuncture*, 1993, Vol. 21, No. 4, p. 313

"Endothelium-dependent Vasodilation in the Brachial Artery is Impaired in Smokers: Effect of Vitamin C," Takeshi Motoyama *et al., American Journal of Physiology: Heart and Circulatory Physiology*, 273: H1644-H1650, 1997

"Epidemiology of Stroke," Oscar Foder, MD, Current Advances in Stroke Symposium, Seattle, WA, June 19, 1986

"Eye Acupuncture," Ricswee Assunta, MD, *The World United Journal for TCM and Acupuncture*, Zuang Ren Publishing Co., Flushing, NY, September, 1997, p. III

"Gait and Balance Dysfunction: A Model of the Interaction of Age and Disease," L. Wolfson, *Neuroscientist,* 2001, Vol. 7, No. 2, p. 178-183

"Heart Disease and Stroke Statistics," American Heart Association, 2004, http://www.americanheart.org

"Hypertension and Stroke," Lawrence Appel, MD, and Rafael Elinas, MD, *The John Hopkins White Papers,* Baltimore, 2005, p. 45-50

"Influence of Different Electro-acupuncture Modes on EEG in Local Cerebral Ischemia in Rats," Jia Qing-shun *et al., International Journal of Clinical Acupuncture,* New York, 2002, Vol. 13, No. 4, p. 283-287

"Influence of Acupuncture on Blood Platelet cAMP, cGMP, Plasma PG12 and TXA2 Contents in Apoplectic Patients," Li Zhong-ren *et al.*, *International Journal of Clinical Acupuncture*, New York, 1990, Vol. 1, No. 2, p. 113-117

"Laser Acupuncture in the Treatment of Paralysis in Stroke Patients: A CT Scan Lesion Site Study," Mararet A. Naeser, *et al.*, *American Journal of Acupuncture*, 1995, Vol. 23, No. 1, p. 13-28

"Morning Blood Pressure May Predict Stroke Risk," P-I News Services, *Seattle Post-Intelligencer*, 2003, March 4, *www.seattlepi.com*

"Moxibustion Treatment of CHD and CVA," Zhang Deng-bu, *International Journal of Clinical Acupuncture*, New York, 1996, Vol. 7, No. 3, p. 285-287

"Observation on Acupuncture Treatment of 322 Cases of Cerebral Infarction and Changes in Serum HDL-C, Fibrinogen, FDP, Hemorrheological Indices etc. During Treatment," Oi L.Y. *et al.*, *International Journal of Clinical Acupuncture*, New York, 1990, Vol. 1, No. 1, p. 39-46

"Ocular Acupuncture Therapy (2)," Peng Jin-shan, *International Journal of Clinical Acupuncture,* New York, 1993, Vol. 4, No. 2, p. 165-170

"Ocular Acupuncture Therapy (1)," Peng Jin-shan, *International Journal of Clinical Acupuncture*, New York, 1993, Vol. 4, No. 1, p. 67-74

"Oral Antioxidant Therapy Improves Endothelial Function in Type 1 but Not Type 2 Diabetes Mellitus," Joshua A. Beckman *et al.*, *American Journal of Physiology: Heart Circulation Physiology*, 2003, 285, p. H2392

"Penn Researchers Add More Evidence To Demonstrate the Role of COX Inhibitors in Heart Disease Risk," Karen Kreeger, University of Pennsylvania Medical Center, Jan. 17, 2005, *http://www.uphs.upenn.edu /news/News_Releases/jan05/COX.htm*

"Prevention of Stroke," Liu Bing-quan, *Sing Tao News*, San Francisco, May 18, 1994, p. B5

"Prevention Conference V: Beyond Secondary Prevention: Identifying the High-Risk Patient for Primary Prevention," Philip Greenland, *et al.*, *Circulation*, 2000; 101, p. 111

"Recommendations and Guidelines Regarding the Preferred Research Protocol for Investigating the Impact of an Optimal Healing Environment on Patients with Hypertension," K. M. Wesa & R. H. Grimm, *The Journal of Alternative and Complementary Medicine,* 2004, 21 Supplement 1, p. S-246

"Scalp Acupuncture in Treating Hemiplegia: Clinical Experience with 24 Cases," Wang Wen-yong, *International Journal of Clinical Acupuncture*, New York, 1996, Vol. 7, No. 4, p. 463-465

"Smoking and the Risk of Hemorrhagic Stroke in Men," T. Kurth *et al.*, *Stroke*, 2003, May; 34(5), p. 1151

"Smoking and Stroke: A Causative Role," Munther Aldoori & Sakhawat Rahman, *BMJ,* 1998; 317, p. 962

"Spread Supplemented with Moderate Doses of Vitamin E and Carotenoids

Reduces Lipid Peroxidation in Healthy, Nonsmoking Adults," Jane E. Pritchard *et al., American Journal of Clinical Nutrition,* November 2003, Vol. 78, No. 5, p. 985

"Stroke Fact Sheet," No author cited, Centers for Disease Control, 1997, *http://www.cdc.gov*

"Stroke," Simeon Margolis, MD, Ph.D. & Robert J. Wityk, MD, *The Johns Hopkins White Papers,* Baltimore, MD, 1998, p. 5

"The Virtues of Greens," Karen Lamphere, *PCC Sound Consumer,* July 2005, No. 83, p. 1

"Tongue Acupuncture (Part I)," Guan Zun-hui, *International Journal of Clinical Acupuncture,* New York, 2000, Vol. 11, No. 1, p. 31-35

"Tongue Acupuncture (Part II)," Guan Zun-hui, *International Journal of Clinical Acupuncture,* New York, 2000, Vol. 11, No. 2, p. 125-128

"Treadmill Aerobic Exercise Training Reduces the Energy Expenditure and Cardiovascular Demands of Hemiparetic Gait in Chronic Stroke Patients: A Preliminary Report," R. F. Macko *et al., Stroke,* American Heart Association, 1997, Vol. 28, No. 2, p. 326-330

"Treating 210 Case of Post Cerebrovascular Disease by First Needling the Healthy Side and then the Affected Side," Li Zhi-xiang *et al., International Journal of Clinical Acupuncture,* New York, 1993, Vol. 4, No. 1, p. 33-34

"Treating A Hidden Cause of Stroke," No author cited, *The John Hopkins Medical Letter,* 1996, March, p. 3

"Trends in Prevalence, Awareness, Treatment, and Control of Hypertension in the United States, 1988-2000," I. Hajjar & T. A. Kotchen, *Journal of the American Medical Association,* 2003; 290, p. 199

"Update on Cholesterol and Red Yeast Rice," *www.wholehealthmd.com*

"Vitamin E May Reduce Risk of Stroke," Richard Benson, 51st Meeting of the American Academy of Neurology, Minneapolis, MN, 1987

Book titles

A Manual Acupuncture, Peter Deadman *et al.,* Eastland Press, Brighton, UK, 1998

Acupuncture: A Comprehensive Text, John O'Connor & Dan Bensky, Eastland Press, Chicago, 1981

Acupuncture Experience Collection, Tian Cong-hua, Science & Technology Articles Publishing Company, Chongqing, 1985

Atlas of Human Anatomy, Frank H. Netter, ICON Learning Systems, place, 1997

Auriculotherapy Manual: Chinese and Western Systems of Ear Acupuncture, 2nd edition, Terry Oleson, Health Care Alternatives, Los Angeles, 1996

Before the Heart Attacks, H. Robert Superko & Laura Tucker, Plume, Penguin Group, New York, 2003

Chinese Herbal Medicine: Formulas & Strategies, Dan Bensky & Randall Barolet, Eastland Press, Seattle, 1986

Chinese Herbal Medicine: Materia Medica, Dan Bensky & Andrew Gamble, Eastland Press, Seattle, 1986

Clinically Oriented Anatomy, Keith L. Moore & Arthur F. Dalley, Lippincott Williams & Wilkins, place, 1999

Human Anatomy & Physiology Laboratory Manual, Elaine N. Marieb, Benjamin/Cummings Science Publishing, place, 1999

Review of Medical Physiology, William F. Ganong, Lange Medical Publications, place, 1981

Compilation of the Abstracts of Acupuncture and Moxibustion Papers, Fong Wan-Kei, The First World Conference of Acupuncture-Moxibustion, Acupuncture Medicine Association of Southern California, date,

Current Medical Diagnosis & Treatment, ed. by Lawrence M. Tierney, Jr. *et al.,* Lange Medical Books/McGraw-Hill, NY, 2002

Dictionary of Chinese Acupuncture, No author cited, Sheep's Publications (HK) Ltd & People's Medical Publishing House, Beijing, 1985

Essentials of Chinese Acupuncture, Beijing College of Traditional Chinese Medicine et al., Foreign Languages Press, Beijing, 1980

Eye Acupuncture Therapy, Peng Jin-shan, Liaoning Science & Technology Publishing, Shenyang, 1990

Eye Acupuncture Therapy, Zhao Xin, trans. by Wang Tai, Academy Press, Beijing, First Edition, 1997

Handbook of Chemistry and Physics, ed. by David R. Lide, CRC Press, 82nd ed., city, 2001-2002

Head Acupuncture, Jiao Shun-fa, trans. by Su Zhi-hong, Shanxi Publishing House, Taiyuan, date

Scalp Needling Therapy, P. S. Yau, Medicine & Health Publishing Co., Hong Kong, 1984

Introduction to English Terminology of Chinese Medicine, Nigel Wiseman & Feng Ye, Paradigm Publications, Brookline, MA, 2002

Prescription for Nutritional Healing, 3rd edition, Phyllis A. Balch & James F. Balch, Avery Publishing, New York, 2000

Scalp Acupuncture and Clinical Cases, Jiao Shun-fa, Foreign Languages Press, Beijing, 1997

Taber's Cyclopedic Medical Dictionary, ed. by Donald Venes, F. A. Davis Company, Philadelphia, 2001

Textbook of Medical Physiology, Arthur C. Guyton, W. B. Saunders Company, place, 1971

The Merck Manual, 17th edition, ed. by Mark H. Beers, MD, Merck Research Laboratories, Whitehouse Station, NJ, 1999

The Nurse's Drug Handbook, Suzanne Loebl *et al.,* Delmar Publishers Inc., place, 1991

The HarperCollins Illustrated Medical Dictionary, Dox, Melloni, & Eisner, HarperCollins Publishers, place, 1993

The Chinese-English Medical Dictionary, ed. by Jin Kui-he, The People's Medical Publishing House, Beijing, 2004

Window of Health: Ocular Diagnosis and Periocular Acupuncture, Hoy Ping Yee Chan, Northwest Institute of Acupuncture & Oriental Medicine, Seattle, WA, 1996

Zhu's Scalp Acupuncture, Zhu Ming-qing, trans. by Dale Chow King & Zheng Yuan-sheng, Eight Dragons Publishing, Hong Kong, 1992

About the Authors

Hoy Ping Yee Chan, a licensed acupuncturist in Washington State, holds a doctoral degree in Oriental Medicine from SAMRA University in Los Angeles. She also holds national board certification as Diplomates of Acupuncture and Chinese Herbology (NCCAOM). Dr. Chan practiced Western medicine in China for 18 years after she graduated from Beijing Medical University. After immigrating to the U.S.A., her focus was to teach and practice acupuncture. Dr. Chan taught at the Northwest Institute of Acupuncture and Oriental Medicine in Seattle for 15 years. Her Chinese Acupuncture Center of North Seattle was one of the first independent acupuncture practices in Washington state when the bill legalizing acupuncture was passed in 1985. Dr. Chan has shared her theories, medical knowledge and health care recommendations during numerous television and newspaper interviews. She has also been a frequent public speaker on issues for community health and continuing education. She has made presentations at acupuncture conferences worldwide in the last twenty years. She is the author of the book *Window of Health: Ocular Diagnosis and Periocular*

Acupuncture. She is one of the first few acupuncturists in the U.S. to know this unique advance micro-acupuncture technique. Clinical research has shown its remarkable effect for treating health conditions, being especially good for stroke in the acute stage. Along with continuing to work in her part-time practice, Dr. Chan feels drawn to share her expanse of knowledge and hard-earned experience with the younger practitioners in our field through books and lectures.

Stanley Sik Chi Chan, M.S., L.Ac, Dipl. Ac. & CH (NCCAOM), was born in Hong Kong and moved to the United States in 1996. He received his Bachelor of Science in Oriental Medicine and Master of Science in Acupuncture and Oriental Medicine at Bastyr University in March 2000 and December 2001 respectively. He is a licensed acupuncturist in Washington State. He has been practicing acupuncture in Seattle since 2002. Mr. Chan has been especially impressed by the effective results of the acupuncture treatments mentioned in the Chinese medical journals he translated for this project. He said, "When I was a student, I learned that acupuncture was effective in treating stroke patients, especially within three months following its onset. Since I lacked clinical experience and knowledge of specific techniques for treating stroke patients, I was excited when Dr. Chan invited me to translate some parts of this book. During my translation work, I was personally fascinated by the bleeding technique of the 12 well points (and its Western medical explanations) used during the acute stage of stroke as well as the variety of techniques for treating post-stroke patients."

Carole Conlon, L.Ac., was in the first graduating class at the Northwest Institute of Acupuncture and Oriental Medicine, becoming an "Acupuncture Therapist" in 1984. Two years later, she sat for and passed exams for national certification in acupuncture through the NCCAOM. Currently practicing in Lynnwood, WA at Spectrum Healing Arts Center, Ms. Conlon specializes in combining traditional Chinese medical theory and acupuncture with several needle-free techniques, including medical dowsing and shamanic healing. Prior to her acupuncture career, Ms. Conlon spent 13 years as a medical technologist working in a variety of hospital settings. She has extensively studied Chinese and Western medicine, Native American shamanism, and a variety of other health and wellness topics and methods. Utilizing the best of each system, she wields them into a powerful yet gentle system of healing and teaching. Because of this interest in education for both self and clients, Ms. Conlon felt impelled to help bring this book on stroke research to fruition. Additionally, Ms. Conlon felt honored to be able to assist Dr. Chan in this endeavor as a way of thanking her for all her contributions during the early years at the Northwest Institute of

Acupuncture and as a leader guiding her class to China for their three month acupuncture internship in Chongqing, Sichuan.

Peter Lau, M.D., a graduate of the University of Santo Tomar-College of Madrona, Phillipines, continued his graduate studies in the U.S. He earned his certification as Diplomate in Internal Medicine and Hematology of the American Board of Internal Medicine and in Blood Banking of the American Board of Pathology. Dr. Lau has spent his professional career in pursuit of excellence and being of service to his patients and the community. He has held faculty positions and served as the medical director of Blood Transfusion Services at the Medical University of Ohio. While he was executive director of the Red Cross Western Regional Blood Center, he established laboratories and programs to support patient care and to advance blood for collection and transfusion in the areas which included bone marrow donor program, stem cell programs, and services to hospitals in certified immunohematology and therapeutic hemapheresis services. He taught students and residents and served as Director of the Blood Transfusion Medicine Fellowship Program. In addition, Dr. Lau has conducted clinical research and has authored over 40 publications. He was honored by the American Red Cross with the prestigious Dr. Charles Drew Award in 2002 and the Presidential Ambassador Award for Cultural Diversity in 1999. He is Professor of Emeritus in Pathology of the Medical College of Ohio. Dr. Lau was exposed to acupuncture when he witnessed his wife's treatments. In his reading of Chinese medical journals, he realized there is much work needed to be done to uncover the scientific basis of this healing art. He jumped at the opportunity of giving Dr.

Chan a hand in Chapter 7 of this book, abstracting and translating the original Chinese to English. It is his hope that this work will promote and continue to unravel the scientific basis of acupuncture.

J. Miranda Ruhland Taylor, a first-generation German-American and native of Rochester, NY, obtained her B.S. degree in biology from Cornell University in Ithaca, NY and her Master degree from the Northwest Institute of Acupuncture and Oriental Medicine. While in school, Miranda searched for an acupuncturist specializing in stroke treatment for a friend and ended up meeting Dr. Chan. After calculating the amount of extra time, money, and energy necessary for rehabilitation after a stroke in the United States (where people wait much too long before getting acupuncture), Miranda decided to focus on prevention with every patient. Her special interest is patient education because compassionate care lies in teaching others how to care for themselves every day. She maintains a private practice, Gesundheit Acupuncture and Herbs, in West Seattle. Her ultimate goal is to work with multi-disciplined (communi-cations, medical, public health, policy, etc.) college students who will encourage high-quality acupuncture in every world community.

Vincent K. Wong was educated in electrical engineering (University of Washington, Seattle, WA) and in biomedical engineering (Case Western Reserve University, Cleveland, OH). After one year in pulmonary research in a hospital in Cleveland, Mr. Wong joined a global conglomerate as an automation engineer. His career evolved and eventually took him to leading IT teams to implement manufacturing and business computer systems in the U.S., Europe, Asia, Australia, and South America. Recently retired, Mr. Wong is devoted to Christian work and the gospel of Jesus Christ. Having been a beneficiary of acupuncture for the infirmity of his lower back, Mr. Wong has long had a desire to be an advocate for Chinese medicine to Western health care professionals and patients at large in whatever ways he can. Hence he contributed a helping hand for the compilation of this book.

General Index

OTHER BOOKS ON CHINESE MEDICINE AVAILABLE FROM:

BLUE POPPY PRESS

5441 Western, Suite 2, Boulder, CO 80301
For ordering 1-800-487-9296 PH. 303\447-8372 FAX 303\245-8362
Email: info@bluepoppy.com Website: www.bluepoppy.com

ACUPOINT POCKET REFERENCE
by Bob Flaws
ISBN 0-936185-93-7

ACUPUNCTURE & IVF
by Lifang Liang
ISBN 0-891845-24-1

ACUPUNCTURE AND MOXIBUSTION
FORMULAS & TREATMENTS
by Cheng Dan-an, trans. by Wu Ming
ISBN 0-936185-68-6

ACUPUNCTURE PHYSICAL MEDICINE: An
Acupuncture Touchpoint Approach to the
Treatment of Chronic Pain, Fatigue, and Stress
Disorders
by Mark Seem
ISBN 1-891845-13-6

AGING & BLOOD STASIS:
A New Approach to TCM Geriatrics
by Yan De-xin
ISBN 0-936185-63-5

A NEW AMERICAN ACUPUNTURE
By Mark Seem
ISBN 0-936185-44-9

BETTER BREAST HEALTH NATURALLY
with CHINESE MEDICINE
by Honora Lee Wolfe & Bob Flaws
ISBN 0-936185-90-2

THE BOOK OF JOOK:
Chinese Medicinal Porridges
by B. Flaws
ISBN 0-936185-60-0

CHANNEL DIVERGENCES
Deeper Pathways of the Web
by Miki Shima and Charles Chase
ISBN 1-891845-15-2

CHINESE MEDICAL OBSTETRICS
by Bob Flaws
ISBN 1-891845-30-6

CHINESE MEDICAL PALMISTRY:
Your Health in Your Hand
by Zong Xiao-fan & Gary Liscum
ISBN 0-936185-64-3

CHINESE MEDICAL PSYCHIATRY
A Textbook and Clinical Manual
by Bob Flaws and James Lake, MD
ISBN 1-845891-17-9

CHINESE MEDICINAL TEAS:
Simple, Proven, Folk Formulas for
Common Diseases & Promoting Health
by Zong Xiao-fan & Gary Liscum
ISBN 0-936185-76-7

CHINESE MEDICINAL WINES & ELIXIRS
by Bob Flaws
ISBN 0-936185-58-9

CHINESE PEDIATRIC MASSAGE THERAPY: A
Parent's & Practitioner's Guide to the Prevention
& Treatment of Childhood Illness
by Fan Ya-li
ISBN 0-936185-54-6

CHINESE SELF-MASSAGE THERAPY:
The Easy Way to Health
by Fan Ya-li
ISBN 0-936185-74-0

THE CLASSIC OF DIFFICULTIES:
A Translation of the Nan Jing
translation by Bob Flaws
ISBN 1-891845-07-1

CLINICAL NEPHROLOGY
IN CHINESE MEDICINE
by Wei Li & David Frierman,
with Ben Luna & Bob Flaws
ISBN 1-891845-23-3

CONTROLLING DIABETES NATURALLY
WITH CHINESE MEDICINE
by Lynn Kuchinski
ISBN 0-936185-06-3

CURING ARTHRITIS NATURALLY WITH
CHINESE MEDICINE
by Douglas Frank & Bob Flaws
ISBN 0-936185-87-2

CURING DEPRESSION NATURALLY WITH
CHINESE MEDICINE
by Rosa Schnyer & Bob Flaws
ISBN 0-936185-94-5

CURING FIBROMYALGIA NATURALLY WITH
CHINESE MEDICINE
by Bob Flaws
ISBN 1-891845-09-8

CURING HAY FEVER NATURALLY WITH
CHINESE MEDICINE
by Bob Flaws
ISBN 0-936185-91-0

CURING HEADACHES NATURALLY WITH
CHINESE MEDICINE
by Bob Flaws
ISBN 0-936185-95-3

CURING IBS NATURALLY WITH CHINESE
MEDICINE
by Jane Bean Oberski
ISBN 1-891845-11-X

CURING INSOMNIA NATURALLY WITH
CHINESE MEDICINE
by Bob Flaws
ISBN 0-936185-86-4

CURING PMS NATURALLY WITH
CHINESE MEDICINE
by Bob Flaws
ISBN 0-936185-85-6

THE DIVINE FARMER'S MATERIA MEDICA
A Translation of the Shen Nong Ben Cao
translation by Yang Shouz-zhong
ISBN 0-936185-96-1

DUI YAO: THE ART OF COMBINING
CHINESE HERBAL MEDICINALS
by Philippe Sionneau
ISBN 0-936185-81-3

ENDOMETRIOSIS, INFERTILITY AND
TRADITIONAL CHINESE MEDICINE:
A Laywoman's Guide
by Bob Flaws
ISBN 0-936185-14-7

THE ESSENCE OF LIU FENG-WU'S
GYNECOLOGY
by Liu Feng-wu, translated by Yang Shou-zhong
ISBN 0-936185-88-0

EXTRA TREATISES BASED ON
INVESTIGATION & INQUIRY:
A Translation of Zhu Dan-xi's Ge Zhi Yu Lun
translation by Yang Shou-zhong
ISBN 0-936185-53-8

FIRE IN THE VALLEY: TCM Diagnosis &
Treatment of Vaginal Diseases
by Bob Flaws
ISBN 0-936185-25-2

FU QING-ZHU'S GYNECOLOGY
trans. by Yang Shou-zhong and Liu Da-wei
ISBN 0-936185-35-X

FULFILLING THE ESSENCE:
A Handbook of Traditional & Contemporary
Treatments for Female Infertility
by Bob Flaws
ISBN 0-936185-48-1

GOLDEN NEEDLE WANG LE-TING: A 20th
Century Master's Approach to Acupuncture
by Yu Hui-chan and Han Fu-ru, trans. by Shuai Xue-
zhong
ISBN 0-936185-789-3

A GUIDE TO GYNECOLOGY
by Ye Heng-yin,
trans. by Bob Flaws and Shuai Xue-zhong
ISBN 1-891845-19-5

A HANDBOOK OF TCM PATTERNS
& TREATMENTS
by Bob Flaws & Daniel Finney
ISBN 0-936185-70-8

A HANDBOOK OF TRADITIONAL
CHINESE DERMATOLOGY
by Liang Jian-hui, trans. by Zhang Ting-liang & Bob
Flaws
ISBN 0-936185-07-4

A HANDBOOK OF TRADITIONAL
CHINESE GYNECOLOGY

by Zhejiang College of TCM, trans. by Zhang Ting-
liang & Bob Flaws
ISBN 0-936185-06-6 (4th edit.)

A HANDBOOK OF CHINESE HEMATOLOGY
by Simon Becker
ISBN 1-891845-16-0

A HANDBOOK OF MENSTRUAL DISEASES IN
CHINESE MEDICINE
by Bob Flaws
ISBN 0-936185-82-1

A HANDBOOK of TCM PEDIATRICS
by Bob Flaws
ISBN 0-936185-72-4

THE HEART & ESSENCE OF DAN-XI'S
METHODS OF TREATMENT
by Xu Dan-xi, trans. by Yang Shou-zhong
ISBN 0-926185-49-X

HERB TOXICITIES & DRUG INTERACTIONS:
A Formula Approach
by Fred Jennes with Bob Flaws
ISBN 1-891845-26-8

IMPERIAL SECRETS OF HEALTH
& LONGEVITY
by Bob Flaws
ISBN 0-936185-51-1

INSIGHTS OF A SENIOR ACUPUNCTURIST
by Miriam Lee
ISBN 0-936185-33-3

INTRODUCTION TO THE USE OF
PROCESSED CHINESE MEDICINALS
by Philippe Sionneau
ISBN 0-936185-62-7

KEEPING YOUR CHILD HEALTHY WITH
CHINESE MEDICINE
by Bob Flaws
ISBN 0-936185-71-6

THE LAKESIDE MASTER'S STUDY
OF THE PULSE
by Li Shi-zhen, trans. by Bob Flaws
ISBN 1-891845-01-2

MASTER HUA'S CLASSIC OF THE
CENTRAL VISCERA
by Hua Tuo, trans. by Yang Shou-zhong
ISBN 0-936185-43-0

MASTER TONG'S ACUPUNCTURE
by Miriam Lee
ISBN 0-926185-37-6

THE MEDICAL I CHING:
Oracle of the Healer Within
by Miki Shima
ISBN 0-936185-38-4

MANAGING MENOPAUSE NATURALLY
with Chinese Medicine
by Honora Lee Wolfe
ISBN 0-936185-98-8

NCCAOM BIO-MEDICINE TEST PREP BOOK:
EXAM PREPARATION & STUDY GUIDE
by Zhong Bai-song
ISBN 978-1-891845-34-9

POINTS FOR PROFIT: The Essential Guide to
Practice Success for Acupuncturists
by Honora Wolfe, Eric Strand & Marilyn Allen
ISBN 1-891845-25-X

THE PULSE CLASSIC:
A Translation of the Mai Jing
by Wang Shu-he, trans. by Yang Shou-zhong
ISBN 0-936185-75-9

SHAOLIN SECRET FORMULAS for Treatment of
External Injuries
by De Chan, trans. by Zhang Ting-liang &
Bob Flaws
ISBN 0-936185-08-2

STATEMENTS OF FACT IN TRADITIONAL
CHINESE MEDICINE
by Bob Flaws
ISBN 0-936185-52-X

STICKING TO THE POINT 1:
A Rational Methodology for the Step by
Step Formulation & Administration of
an Acupuncture Treatment
by Bob Flaws
ISBN 0-936185-17-1

STICKING TO THE POINT 2:
A Study of Acupuncture & Moxibustion
Formulas and Strategies
by Bob Flaws
ISBN 0-936185-97-X

A STUDY OF DAOIST ACUPUNCTURE &
MOXIBUSTION
by Liu Zheng-cai
ISBN 1-891845-08-X

THE SUCCESSFUL CHINESE HERBALIST
by Bob Flaws and Honora Lee Wolfe
ISBN 1-891845-29-2

THE SYSTEMATIC CLASSIC OF
ACUPUNCTURE & MOXIBUSTION
A translation of the Jia Yi Jing
by Huang-fu Mi, trans. by Yang Shou-zhong & Charles
Chace
ISBN 0-936185-29-5

THE TAO OF HEALTHY EATING
ACCORDING TO CHINESE MEDICINE
by Bob Flaws
ISBN 0-936185-92-9

TEACH YOURSELF TO READ MODERN
MEDICAL CHINESE
by Bob Flaws
ISBN 0-936185-99-6

TREATING PEDIATRIC BED-WETTING WITH
ACUPUNCTURE & CHINESE MEDICINE
by Robert Helmer
ISBN 978-1-891845-33-0

THE TREATMENT OF CARDIOVASCULAR
DISEASES WITH CHINESE MEDICINE
by Simon Becker, Bob Flaws &
Robert Casañas, MD
ISBN 978-1-891845-27-6

THE TREATMENT OF DIABETES
MELLITUS WITH CHINESE MEDICINE
by Bob Flaws, Lynn Kuchinski &
Robert Casañas, M.D.
ISBN 1-891845-21-7

THE TREATMENT OF DISEASE IN TCM, Vol. 1:
Diseases of the Head & Face, Including Mental &
Emotional Disorders
by Philippe Sionneau & Lü Gang
ISBN 0-936185-69-4

THE TREATMENT OF DISEASE IN TCM, Vol. II:
Diseases of the Eyes, Ears, Nose, & Throat
by Sionneau & Lü
ISBN 0-936185-69-4

THE TREATMENT OF DISEASE, Vol. III: Diseases
of the Mouth, Lips, Tongue,
Teeth & Gums
by Sionneau & Lü
ISBN 0-936185-79-1

THE TREATMENT OF DISEASE, Vol IV: Diseases
of the Neck, Shoulders,
Back, & Limbs
by Philippe Sionneau & Lü Gang
ISBN 0-936185-89-9

THE TREATMENT OF DISEASE, Vol V: Diseases
of the Chest & Abdomen
by Philippe Sionneau & Lü Gang
ISBN 1-891845-02-0

THE TREATMENT OF DISEASE, Vol VI: Diseases
of the Urogential System
& Proctology
by Philippe Sionneau & Lü Gang
ISBN 1-891845-05-5

THE TREATMENT OF DISEASE, Vol VII: General
Symptoms
by Philippe Sionneau & Lü Gang
ISBN 1-891845-14-4

THE TREATMENT OF EXTERNAL
DISEASES WITH ACUPUNCTURE
& MOXIBUSTION
by Yan Cui-lan and Zhu Yun-long, trans. by Yang Shou-
zhong
ISBN 0-936185-80-5

THE TREATMENT OF MODERN
WESTERN MEDICAL DISEASES
WITH CHINESE MEDICINE
by Bob Flaws & Philippe Sionneau
ISBN 1-891845-20-9

THE TREATMENT OF DIABETES
MELLITUS WITH CHINESE MEDICINE
by Bob Flaws, Lynn Kuchinski
& Robert Casañas, MD
ISBN 1-891845-21-7

UNDERSTANDING THE DIFFICULT PATIENT: A
Guide for Practitioners of Oriental Medicine
by Nancy Bilello, RN, L.ac.
ISBN 1-891845-32-2

70 ESSENTIAL CHINESE
HERBAL FORMULAS
by Bob Flaws
ISBN 0-936185-59-7

160 ESSENTIAL CHINESE HERBAL PATENT
MEDICINES
by Bob Flaws
ISBN 1-891945-12-8

630 QUESTIONS & ANSWERS ABOUT
CHINESE HERBAL MEDICINE:
A Workbook & Study Guide
by Bob Flaws
ISBN 1-891845-04-7

230 ESSENTIAL CHINESE MEDICINALS
by Bob Flaws
ISBN 1-891845-03-9

750 QUESTIONS & ANSWERS ABOUT
ACUPUNCTURE
Exam Preparation & Study Guide
by Fred Jennes
ISBN 1-891845-22-5